Language Pangs

Language Pangs

On Pain and the Origin of Language

ILIT FERBER

OXFORD
UNIVERSITY PRESS

OXFORD
UNIVERSITY PRESS

Oxford University Press is a department of the University of Oxford. It furthers the University's objective of excellence in research, scholarship, and education by publishing worldwide. Oxford is a registered trade mark of Oxford University Press in the UK and certain other countries.

Published in the United States of America by Oxford University Press
198 Madison Avenue, New York, NY 10016, United States of America.

CIP data is on file at the Library of Congress
ISBN 978–0–19–005386–4

1 3 5 7 9 8 6 4 2

Printed by Sheridan Books, Inc., United States of America

In memoriam: Werner Hamacher

CONTENTS

ACKNOWLEDGMENTS

The experience of pain is all about isolation, separation, and the singular, inescapable feeling of oneself. It is, in many senses, about being alone. But pain, and in this case, writing about it, is also about creating an intimacy with others, turning toward them, listening and being listened to. It is about the unique way in which the world is sometimes and surprisingly, attentive to you.

I am thankful to all those who have given their attention to this project, supported and inspired it. I am grateful to Eli Friedlander for the invaluable and long-standing philosophical dialogue and for his unwavering friendship; to Andrew Benjamin, Adam Lipszic, and Ori Rotlevy who read parts of the many transformations of this book, for their careful reading and helpful suggestions; María del Rosario Acosta López and Peter Fenves for their comments and suggestions on the final version of the book; Hagi Kenaan for his interest and support throughout the years; Omer Michaelis, my wonderful research assistant, for his indispensable help and insightful suggestions; Orna Harari and Shraon Weisser for their help with the Greek; Arnd Wedemeyer for introducing Herder to me many years ago; Lucy Randall of Oxford University Press for her encouragement and belief in the project; Hannah Doyle and Christina Nisha Paul, also of Oxford University Press, for their help in bringing the book to completion; my students from the philosophy department of Tel-Aviv University for their patience and difficult questions. I would also like to thank some of my most avid interlocuters: Michal Grover-Friedlander, Moshe Halbertal, Vivian Liska, Mirjam Hadar, Michael W. Jennings, Aïcha Liviana-Messina, Menachem Lorberboim, Josi Mali, Tamar Mayer, Hindy Najman, Dana Olmert, Freddie Rokem, Ruth Ronen, Caroline Sauter, Nassima Sahraoui, and Galili Shahar, for their interest and encouraging support.

I am grateful to my family for their love that is and always was everything to me. Most of all, I thank my husband Roy for his support and for being there for me in all the happy as well as painful moments that accompanied my writing.

Without his love this book would not have been possible. To my children who listened to the story of Philoctetes at bedtime so many times: I thank Ori for our conversations and her beautiful questions, Adam for his unique sensitivity and ability to make me laugh also in painful moments, and Yotam whose insights about empathy accompany this book.

The work was written amid many conversations with Werner Hamacher. I am grateful for his attention, generosity, and belief in the project. Werner passed away just a few months before the manuscript was completed and our last meeting was devoted to discussing its final details. It is a great sadness that he did not live to see it in print. This book is dedicated to him.

ABBREVIATIONS

The list below provides abbreviations for frequently cited works throughout the text. Abbreviations for other works not on this list are given in the endnotes at the first mention of the work being cited.

WORK BY CAVELL

Acknow.	"Knowing and Acknowledging." In *Must We Mean What We Say?*, 238–266. Cambridge University Press, 1976.

WORKS BY HEIDEGGER

Seminar	*On the Essence of Language: The Metaphysics of Language and the Essencing of the Word. Concerning Herder's Treatise on the Origin of Language*, trans. Wanda Torres Gregory and Yvonna Unna. State University of New York Press, 2004.
Seminar-N	Heidegger's notes.
Seminar-T	Student transcripts.
WS	*Vom Wesen der Sprache: Die Metaphysik der Sprache und die Wesung des Wortes. Zu Herders Abhandlung "Über den Ursprung der Sprache."* In *Gesamtausgabe*, vol. 85., ed. Ingrid Schüßler. Vittorio Klostermann GmbH, 1999.

WORKS BY HERDER

AS	*Abhandlung über den Ursprung der Sprache*. In *Werke*: Bd. 1: Frühe Schriften 1764–1772, ed. Urich Gaier, 697–810. Deutscher Klassiker Verlag, 1985.
Treatise	"Treatise on the Origin of Language." In *Philosophical Writings*, trans. and ed. Michael N. Forster, 65–164. Cambridge University Press, 2002.

VERSIONS OF *PHILOCTETES*

Gide, Philoc.	André Gide. "Philoctetes; or, the Treatise on Three Ethics." In *Philoctetes and the Fall of Troy: Documents, Iconography, Interpretations*, ed. and trans. Oscar Mandel, 158–178. University of Nebraska Press, 1981.
Herder, Philoc.	Johann Gottfried Herder. "Philoktetes: Szenen mit Gesang." In *Nachlaß veröffentlicht, Sämmtliche Werke*. [Abt.] Zur schönen Literatur und Kunst 6. Theil, ed. J. G. Herder, 113–126. Cotta, 1806.
Müller, Philoc.	Heiner Müller. "Philoctetes." In *Philoctetes and the Fall of Troy*, trans. Oscar Mandel in collaboration with Maria Kelsen Feder, 222–250. University of Nebraska Press, 1981.
Sophocles, Philoc.	Sophocles. *Philoctetes*. trans. Hugh Lloyd-Jones. Loeb Classical Library. Harvard University Press, 1998.

WORK BY ROUSSEAU

Essay	"Essay on the Origin of Languages." In *Essay on the Origin of Languages and Writings Related to Music* (*Collected Writings of Rousseau*, vol. 7), trans. and ed. John T. Scott, 247–299. University Press of New England, 1998.

Language Pangs

1

On Pain and the Origin of Language

At first glance, it seems evident that language and pain have entirely different—if not opposing—structures. Paradigmatic of the utterly private, pain, when it invades our bodies, separates us from anyone who is not subject to its overwhelming vehemence. From the linguistic perspective, pain marks an even deeper divide between the sufferer and the world: completely inaccessible and invisible to anyone other than the person who experiences it, pain is fundamentally excluded from articulate and communicative linguistic expression. Pain is therefore usually regarded as an experience that cannot be fully expressed in language, something we can never entirely communicate or share with others. Its unmediated nature tends to be deemed private, inasmuch as any attempt to articulate it publicly is doomed to fail. Along these lines, language seems to be everything that pain is not. Its underlying principles are those of shareability, communication, and various forms of the self's extension into the world and toward others.

Regardless of our theoretical orientation toward language—whether analytical, continental, or logical—this configuration of language, and the various ways by which it refers, represents, expresses, and communicates, is common to them all. Language not only challenges the private and solipsistic structure of pain, but it also constitutes itself as inherently distinct from everything that is of-the-body, somatic, or nonsymbolic. In this sense, physical pain and the body as such must be overcome in order for language to emerge. If the emergence of language marks humans' departure from the bestial, then the violence and intensity of cries of pain are precisely what can turn us back into animals, or at least—momentarily—expose the animality that saturates our linguistic being.

Language Pangs challenges these already familiar conceptions and proposes a reconsideration of the relationship between pain and language in terms of an essential interconnectedness rather than the common exclusive opposition. My premise is both that we cannot truly penetrate the experience of pain without taking account of its inherent relation to language, and, vice versa, that the nature of language essentially depends on our understanding of its inherent relationship with pain. I question the assumption that the experience of pain puts a basic limit to our linguistic abilities, neutralizing us as linguistic beings. On the contrary, the exploration of the nature and origins of language reveals a very strong kinship to pain. It is therefore necessary to shift away from considering this relationship in terms of essential rivalry and opposition and turn toward a notion of inherent interconnection and profound intimacy between pain and language, an abiding intimacy. Although it might be irrefutable that in states of extreme pain, language seems to crumble or collapse, depriving us of words, considering this characterization in itself is problematic and partial, stemming perhaps from the way in which pain and language are conceptualized and defined in the first place.

Although I concentrate mainly on physical and not psychic pain or suffering, my discussion is not limited to the physical aspects and implications of pain (if it is at all possible to treat pain as having merely physical implications). The prevalent use of the word "pain" in the context of mental suffering (the pain of loss, longing, or even love) reveals the kinship between physical and mental pain. It is moreover difficult, perhaps impossible, to find philosophical discussions of physical pain that do not "spill over" into its mental, psychological effects. Discussions that remain within the boundaries of the merely physical aspects of pain are, generally speaking, disciplinary and therefore rather limited (medical discussions for instance). I am interested in the ways in which the experience of pain affects (destroying as well as constituting) our sense of being and self, our experience of others and of the world as such, and finally, our linguistic existence. My understanding of suffering is not limited to its interpretation as what is sometimes treated, in categories of the philosophy of mind, as a "judgement" of pain, or even as one of pain's "aspects." In my discussion, pain is not "transformed" into something else that transcends the merely physical, nor is pain viewed, here, as a mere "cause" of mental suffering. I characterize the experience of pain as an experience of boundaries, by its being *on* the boundary: always between the physical and psychic, both internal and external, undifferentiated from our very identity but at the same time emerging as our utmost negation.

There is therefore a double register at play in my use of the term "pain." Even when I delve into a detailed phenomenology of the experience of physical or mental pain, what I refer to is not pain as a discrete event or feeling. I will move, in this sense, rather freely between physical pain, mental suffering, and a more general sense of suffering. Pain is so important precisely because of its unmatched ability to transcend itself, to be suggestive of so much more than a headache or open wound. Its significance is fully achieved when, to use Cioran's beautiful words, "wounds cease to be mere outer manifestations without deep complications and begin to participate in the essence of your being."[1] I regard pain, therefore, as a philosophical figure. This, however, should not remove pain from its bodily experience and, more generally put, its somatic setting and implications. Pain's uniqueness inheres precisely in the distinct way in which it allows for this intersection between the most basic, coarse bodily sensation, on the one hand, and its philosophical purport, on the other. These implications, as I will show, are not invariably known or cognitively perceived, but they are nevertheless deeply felt. The experience of extreme pain is always coupled with an inherent transcendence of its physical aspect to an encounter with and redefinition of the conditions of experience as such: an experience not only of the body in pain, but also and foremost, a sense of our very being, world, and language—having opened up in ways that are not open to us otherwise, that is, without pain.

Although pain's revelatory power is abundant, this book concentrates on one crucial dimension enfolded in the experience of pain, namely, language and expression. Pain is famously discussed as a force utterly destructive to language; it is conceived as undermining our ability to communicate our suffering, threatening the very possibility of our relationship to other human beings. Pain's intensity has undeniably crucial bearing on our language and communicative abilities but it would be problematically restrictive, to say the least, to view these effects as merely destructive, robbing us of our very humanity and the possibility to feel for others. This book's approach suggests a different view on their relationship. When pain encounters language it tears it apart, and in doing so its very essence is laid bare. Importantly—and pain's uniqueness, over and beyond that of other feelings or emotions, is located here—it reveals language's innermost being as inseparable from bodily feeling, suffering, and sympathy. It is in its intercourse with pain that language can be thought of as transcending the binaries of human and animal, inside and outside, man and object.

The encounter between pain and language is deemed destructive only insofar as we conceive of language as a mere instrument with which we refer to pain or try to communicate it—say something *about* it. When we consider language, rather, as an expressive apparatus stretching beyond this merely propositional structure, a variety of ways emerge in which pain encapsulates the very conditions of possibility of expression and language.[2] Pain is, therefore, not only about the failure or collapse of language. It is also, and more powerfully, a vigorous force demanding expression. From this point of view, pain does not work against language; instead, it realizes its inclination and drive to express and gets language to work. Pain, therefore, manifests something of the strength of language, its boundlessness rather than weakness or collapse; it brings forth the possibilities of language as such, the very conditions that make it what it is.

A Phenomenology of Pain

The intensity of the experience of extreme pain is almost unmatched. Pain seems to invade us like an omnipotent, invincible force, overtaking us completely, engulfing us. Pain is not simply something we "have" or "feel"; it does not merely "color" our world or our physical experience. It soon becomes the dominant mode of our very being. We experience pain as an all-consuming force, embracing and devouring us at the same time. When it strikes, we do not merely undergo an agonizing bodily sensation: pain directly affects our very sense of self. Instead of feeling ourselves *in* pain, we *become* our pain, united with it so that there is nothing but pain. With the emergence of pain, our most basic sense of self is violated, posing a fundamental challenge to our fragile, composite existence as our unity of self is utterly devastated.[3] It is in this sense that any understanding of pain as a physical, determinate, and well-defined "event" is insubstantial.

Pain harbors the potential of transfiguring our very being. Living in the reality of intense pain (whether acute or chronic, physical or psychological) is neither an event nor a state; it is not even a quality of our customary, familiar existence. The experience of pain violently thrusts us into a unique existential state in which it becomes the consummate foundation of our very being, its organizing principle. Even when pain is chronic, a pain that is always there but never acute or intense, our mode of being is constituted by it, profoundly marked and distinguished by its ever-present constraint. About this, Emily Dickinson writes that "Pain—has an Element of Blank—/It cannot recollect/When it begun—Or if there were/A time when it was not—/It has no Future—but itself—/Its Infinite contain/Its Past—enlightened to perceive/New Periods—Of Pain."[4] For Dickinson, admitting pain enforces acceptance of its rule over time and space, over us and our world. There is nothing but pain: neither past nor future, and especially no reference point to "when it is not." This is yet another of pain's hallmarks: it completely fills us, condensing our identity, temporal experience, and relationship to everything outside us and outside it. And everything indeed is outside it. There is nothing but pain.

Pain forces itself on us as our one and only center, the crux of our being. It is not only the body that becomes dominated by it: pain seems to draw and gather every inch of our attention and energy into its whirlpool motion. At first, we feel as if pain, like an uninvited guest, enters from the outside, invading us, striking with all its force until we disintegrate. This quality of foreignness, however, turns out to be not that simple. Given the relentless power of its grip, pain has a transformative impact, which also affects our initial relation to it, especially the sense of its foreignness. Pain is thus transfigured: appearing at first as though it was external, an alien "agency" that confronts us, it almost unnoticeably becomes uniquely internal and intimate. Once it has become an inseparable part of us, we cannot remove ourselves from pain and its intensity even if we wanted nothing more dearly: we might as well choose to withdraw from our very selves.[5]

Enduring pain is indeed an experience of utter privacy and isolation: we experience our pains alone. The totality with which pain isolates us is not only singular insofar as it completely embeds us; it also uniquely reconstitutes, perhaps even re-creates, the foundations of our relationship to everything else: self, body, world, and language. The experience of utter separation and segregation so inherent to pain opens a chasm between the before and after of pain. It is now the sufferer alone, confronting himself or herself in a wholly different manner: in the utter absence of anything *but* pain—a bare, sensitive body, with nothing external to refer to, feel for, or relate to. The overwhelming retreat that pain forces on us compels us to face pain, from a minimal distance, from within an enclosed space that permits no withdrawal.

The conception of pain as isolating can also be found in psychoanalytic theory, first and foremost in Freud's early work.[6] Although he rarely discusses physical pain in his works ("We know very little about pain," he writes),[7] Freud provides us with a suggestive understanding of physical pain in terms of a solipsistic retreat, a withdrawal from the world: being in pain, he writes, is always coupled with a fundamental relinquishing of interest in the outside world, in everything that does not concern our suffering.[8] He perceptively describes pain as an "*in-drawing*" occurring in the internal, mental sphere, an "*internal haemorrhage*," operating just like a wound.[9] With the metaphor of the internal, bleeding wound, Freud offers us an economic model of the total withdrawal that is so distinctive of physical pain.[10] Pain literally sucks us in, preventing us from being invested in anything else but pain. The excessive nature of pain is coupled here with the impoverishment so characteristic of melancholic withdrawal from the world: the first is too much, the other, barely enough.[11]

Among the many facets and implications of pain's breach, standing out is its ability to devastate any possibility we have to respond to it or to act against it. Whereas one of the foundations of subjectivity (at least in its modern conception) refers to agency, when we are in pain we face ourselves as downright passive.[12] Pain's inexorable demand for total submission leaves us defenseless. But this powerful clench of pain is not simply overwhelming; it is, more importantly, an experience from which we cannot withdraw, a state from which there is no refuge. Emmanuel Levinas' description of physical pain is especially suggestive here: "Physical suffering, in all its degrees entails the impossibility of detaching oneself from the instance of existence. It is the very irremissibility of being [l'être]. The content of suffering merges with the impossibility of detaching oneself from suffering. . . . The whole acuity of suffering lies in this impossibility of retreat. . . . In this sense suffering is the impossibility of nothingness."[13]

Unable to act against pain, we are forced to submit to it, take it upon ourselves, and become one with it. This submission, however, also means that we cannot absorb the experience of pain into our world and existence by assuming it into a meaningful structure. The fundamental interruption exercised by pain, in other words, is not merely and discretely experienced in the body of the suffering individual but affects his or her most basic ability to *signify* pain. Pain is therefore often experienced and conceived of as unintelligible, constantly challenging our very ability to assimilate and integrate it in our lives.

The way in which pain strikes, undermines, and even rejects the possibility of maintaining a fixed structure of sense or meaning profoundly interferes with our ability to synthesize. This is not because of, as Levinas explains, the excessive intensity of the experience of pain, its "too muchness"; it is, rather, an excess that penetrates the dimensions of meaning which, when not suffering, we take to be open to us. There is, then, a fundamental denial of meaning that is inherent to pain, a unique form of an unbearable experience. Levinas points out the paradoxical coexistence of the unbearable nature of pain with the fact that there is simply no question of *not* bearing it. That is, while we are compelled to bear our pain, it is at the same time the epitome of the fundamentally unbearable.[14] Blanchot follows a similar line when he characterizes physical suffering as what we can neither suffer nor cease to suffer, an experience that places us at time's point of suspension, where the present is an ongoing moment, without either future or projection, "an impassable infinite, the infinite of suffering."[15] Jean Améry's description of his harrowing experiences in the Nazi camps reveals a similar approach when he refers to the senselessness of any attempt to describe his experiences of pain since "qualities of feelings are as incomprehensible as they are indescribable."[16] For Améry it is not enough to point at the disintegration of language; there is a more profound understanding here that the collapse of linguistic capabilities marks a deeper collapse: that of the logical possibility of our very existence.

There is a plethora of literary works that look at the fundamental discordance between pain and our ability to express it, all pointing at language's collapse in the face of intense pain.[17] Pain has often been described as a watertight barrier to language, in front of which the latter slowly, or at times suddenly, crumbles. This failure is felt all the more strongly because the experience of intense pain is so compellingly tied to the need to express it. Pain seems to demand expression, as if internally pressing us to voice it, insisting that it be poured out in facial expressions, bodily contortions, sounds, and cries. It seems then rather plausible to argue that along the spectrum of feelings and sensations, pain most forcefully and immediately demands its own expression, while it is distinctly when we are in pain that we so markedly fail to do so. The irreconcilable nature of these two characteristics—the striving toward expression and the impossibility of actualizing it—is what makes physical pain stand out as unique. It marks the height of our yearning to express but at the same time confronts us with the impossibility of doing so. When pain strikes, there is no room for words, only howls. Language can function again only when the overwhelming effect of pain is replaced by its faint memory.

The opposition between pain and language is frequently portrayed in terms of the impotence of language in its encounter with the ferocity of pain. Virginia Woolf famously writes that "English, which can express the thoughts of Hamlet and the tragedy of Lear, has no words for the shiver and the headache . . . but let a sufferer try to describe a pain in his head to a doctor and language at once runs dry. He is forced to coin words himself, and, taking his pain in one hand, and a lump of pure sound in the other . . . so to crush them together that a brand new word in the end drops out."[18] Elsewhere she observes that "for pain words are lacking. There should be cries, cracks, fissures, whiteness passing over chintz covers, interference with the sense of time, of space."[19] What is so striking for Woolf is the disparity between the richness and profusion of language's ability to express extremely complex thoughts and feelings and its collapse in the face of pain. Linguistic plentitude runs dry when one finds no words for a shiver or headache—that is, for the most basic, everyday experiences. For these, there are only sounds and cries, "a lump of pure sound," but no words, let alone a communicative comprehensive account.

As cogent and telling as it is, this description presents us with a difficulty. We feel that we know what pain is: we have all experienced it in one way or another, whether a suffocating all-encompassing pain induced by violence, or a mere, passing headache. Insofar as we are human, we are sensitive to pain and subject to its power. We know the suffering inherent to it at first hand; we have felt its constraints and have all, to some extent, been lost for words in the face of intense pain. It is by instinct, physical as well as psychological, that we fight against pain, make every effort to avoid it, or if there is no other option, cure it or make it go away. Thus we instantly connect to philosophical, and especially literary, descriptions of how the experience of pain feels and what it causes: it is as if these put words to what we deeply but wordlessly know. However, our immediate sense of recognition of these phenomenological descriptions all too often tempts us to assume they capture something of the singular nature, heart, and depth of pain. I use the word "temptation" to draw attention to how this sense of recognition may also narrow down our perspective on the issue at hand, revealing it exclusively under the narrow beam of its stark, dangerously blinding light.

The Two Paradigms

The recent literature on pain clarifies something about this temptation. This can be demonstrated by way of two primary intuitions prevalent in the literature about pain. First, the emphasis on the destructive nature of pain: pain destroys our bodies, souls, linguistic abilities, and the possibility to communicate with others. Second, pain isolates us, opening up an unbridgeable gap between the experience of our own suffering and everything else: world, objects, others. It would be safe to say that these two postulates have by now crystallized into two key paradigms that have become almost inextricable from the way we think about pain, even feel it. According to the first paradigm, pain is fundamentally characterized by its *destructiveness*; according to the second, pain is violently *isolating*, turning us into enclosed, solipsistic entities. Pain dismantles our world and being and our ability to actively exercise our subjectivity, not only because it literally destroys our bodily integrity, but more important, as a consequence of its impact on our linguistic, communicative capabilities, it renders them virtually powerless.[20]

Both paradigms play a central role in Elaine Scarry's acclaimed *The Body in Pain*. Although since its publication in 1985, Scarry's work has become a reference point for any examination of pain, her book suffers from some weaknesses sometimes found pioneering research. Among the first books to emphasize the far-reaching political implications of the experience of pain and violence, it presents a fundamentally partial and biased account that fails to do justice to her subject, the body in pain.[21] The main reason for this, I assume, is that Scarry's book focuses on a discussion of war and torture, that is, extreme cases of pain inflicted in the context of political enmity. For these cases, Scarry's analysis is no doubt valid,[22] but it leaves out many other contexts, degrees, and configurations of pain. That said, I will refer to Scarry in order to establish my argument for the existence of the two paradigmatic portrayals of pain (which she largely developed), while presenting her position with a critical eye.

Although her discussion claims to address both the "making" as well as the "unmaking" of the world when it is affected by pain—Scarry emphasizes the second aspect, namely, the ways in which pain shatters and destroys the world and subjectivity as we know it. Scarry skillfully draws a picture of a fierce confrontation between pain and, generally speaking, human existence (or the world), with pain featuring as an overwhelming, destructive force. Thus Scarry conceives of pain as a "pure physical experience of negation, an immediate sensory rendering of 'against,'" to the point of there being a "simple and absolute incompatibility of pain and the world."[23] But even more distinctive about Scarry's account is her emphasis on the metaphoric language we usually use when describing pain as a form of agency, as though it attacked us intentionally and purposefully acted upon us. Her rhetoric is consequently dominated by metaphors that support such a notion of pain: "It feels as though a hammer is coming down on my spine"—where there is no concrete hammer; or "It feels as if my arm is broken at each joint and the jagged ends are sticking through the skin even where the bones of the arms are intact and the surface of the skin is unbroken,"[24] and so forth. Extreme physical pain, according to Scarry, "does not simply resist language but actively destroys it" and is "monolithically consistent in its assault on language."[25]

Susan Sontag analyzed the rhetoric and imagery of medical accounts of pain, identifying images comparable to those Scarry uses. Sontag demonstrates that the dominant metaphors of illness and pain are often borrowed from the language of warfare. She shows, for instance, that cancer is often described as "the barbarian within"; cancer cells do not simply multiply but are "invasive,"[26] and the disease and its effects are being "magnified and projected into a metaphor for the biggest enemy . . . a form of demonic possession."[27] Sontag continues to demonstrate that the descriptions of medical treatments "fighting" pain and disease use similarly military language: "radiotherapy uses the metaphors of aerial warfare; patients are 'bombarded' with toxic rays. And chemotherapy is chemical warfare, using poisons."[28] These characterizations of disease and the pain that accompanies it as obstructive enemies not only depict the representatives of the medical system as salvaging benefactors struggling against pain and vanquishing it, but also and perhaps foremost, they portray pain as a menacing threat, our worst enemy. Pain invades our bodies and lives, shatters our linguistic abilities, and accomplishes the absolute, perfect disruption. Depleting language, pain takes an antagonistic, aversive role and eventually triumphs by rendering itself, in Scarry's terminology, "unshareable": "Whatever pain achieves," she writes, "it achieves in part through its unsharability, and it ensures this unsharability through its resistance to language."[29] In order to make sense of this argument, which is perhaps the cornerstone of her book, it is necessary to closely consider some of Scarry's other key points.

According to Scarry, most of our states of consciousness refer to external objects (we love *someone*, fear *something*, are ambivalent *about* something, etc.). This configuration is interrupted, she writes, "when, moving through the human interior, one at last reached physical pain, for physical pain—unlike any other state of consciousness—has no referential content. It is not *of* or *for* anything. It is precisely because it takes no object that it, more than any other phenomenon, resists objectification in language."[30] Pain, then, may have an objective reason (it can be brought about by illness or an armed attack), but this does not mean that the experience of pain itself has a referential structure. It is obvious where Scarry wants to take her argument: since it has no object (i.e., it is not about or for something) pain has no objective, public presence. It remains private and cannot thus be configured into an objective, referential structure that can be shared with others. Pain is unsharable in principle, doomed to an everlasting, profound privacy which renders it nonlinguistic. Hannah Arendt considers similar ideas in a political context, arguing that pain deprives us of the possibility to reach out from the private to the public realm. This is not only because of our inability to transform its utter privacy into content suitable for public discourse but also because it violently detaches us from anything we can call a world. If we conceive of reality as a world we all see and hear concomitantly, Arendt argues, then pain marks the passage into a shadowy, uncertain form of existence and is hence automatically deemed a "private matter."[31]

This has far-reaching implications: primarily it means that pain is a threat to our very humanity. If being human is understood as having a language, being a speaking creature, and pain is the experience that destroys language, then pain is constituted, in Scarry's account, as obliterating the very possibility of our being human. This deprivation of humanity is twofold: first, those *in pain* are bereft of their humanity because they are deprived of their language—the very foundation of their humanity; and second, those *witnessing pain* become inhuman by contagion, since in the encounter with the other's pain, they cannot fundamentally feel empathy. In both cases, the deprivation of humanity is inherently connected with a deprivation of language. In Scarry's account, extreme pain not only destroys language but also brings about "an immediate reversion to a state anterior to language, to the sounds and cries a human being makes before language is learned."[32] When in pain, man loses his every shred of humanity and immediately and fundamentally regresses to literal infantility, left with his mere bodily, animal constituents. Pain deprives us of what makes us human.

Here the two aforementioned paradigms—destructiveness and isolation—come together. Pain is world-destroying, to use Scarry's term, not only because it destroys the suffering subject's capabilities, the ones that constitute his or her humanity, but first and foremost, since it destroys the possibility of the sufferer's relationships with others. The shattering of pain's referential structure grounds Scarry's argument that there is a fundamental incongruence between one's own pain and the pain of others: pain's nonreferential structure renders it unsharable, opening up the chasm between one's own pain and the pain of the other. Using metaphors of geographical distance, Scarry compares the pain of others to "some deep subterranean fact, belonging to an invisible geography that, however portentous, has no reality because it has not yet manifested itself on the visible surface of the earth." She describes the painful events taking place in another's body as "vaguely alarming yet unreal, laden with consequence yet evaporating before the mind because not available to sensory confirmation . . . and the pains occurring in other people's bodies flicker before the mind, then disappear."[33] To the sufferer, pain is immediately and "effortlessly" grasped, without a trace of doubt. For the one witnessing another's suffering, Scarry claims, it is precisely the opposite: the unreality, even denial of the other's pain. This chasm marks the paradoxical nature of pain, an experience we cannot deny and cannot confirm, at one and the same time.[34]

The problematic nature of the convergence between destructiveness and isolation, the two paradigms of pain, emerges most clearly when we take into account Scarry's emphasis on the essential discrepancy between our own pain and the pains of others. She grounds her argument in a strictly epistemological perspective, establishing the threatening gap enforced by pain's paradoxical nature, in terms of the essential disparity between the certainty we have of our own pains and the inevitable doubt we feel toward other people's pains. This narrow definition is the heart of what the field of the Philosophy of Mind describes as "the problem of other minds." This problem is premised on the discrepancy between the knowledge we have of our own pain, knowledge that is immediate and certain beyond doubt, and any knowledge we have of other people's pain, which is of necessity indirect and inherently open to doubt.[35] To follow Thomas Nagel's famous formulation of the problem (which in turn follows Wittgenstein), the crux of the problem has to do with the difference between *feeling* one's pain and *knowing* (or not knowing) the pain of another person. Nagel thus importantly presents the problem of other minds as a strictly epistemological problem. Since pain can only be recognized by introspection (and never knowledge, since I cannot know my own pain, only feel it) and is essentially based on first-person claim knowledge, we can never have substantial enough grounds for knowing, let alone experiencing, other people's pain. Considering the relationship between our own pain and the pain of others solely in terms of knowledge constitutes an incomplete, limited account of the problem.[36]

Since we cannot enter other people's minds, we are left with the only thing that is publicly available: the external, behavioral expressions produced by those in pain. This leads, in the discussion of the "problem of other minds," to what is standardly called the "argument from analogy." According to this argument, because we have access only to our own pain, we use our own case as a point of reference and treat other people's pain as analogous to our own. Insofar as we are all human, the similarity of our pain is inferred. The weakness here is clear: there is no firm basis to argue for correlation; we can never have more than an assumption, and it follows that we can never have firm grounds for arguing that someone else is indeed in pain. We are always and necessarily certain of our own pain, and inherently in doubt regarding the pain of others. Moreover, the structure of the argument reinforces the problem: a relationship based on analogy necessarily presupposes separation. Even from this short and basic account of the crux of the problem of other minds, it is already clear how its epistemological slant paves the way for what appears to be a convincing connection between the experience of pain, our relationship to others, and radical skepticism.[37]

Pain and Language

The discrepancy between pain's unmatched intensity and urgency and the inability to thrust it into language is indeed one of its deepest distinguishing marks. It is irrefutable that in states of extreme pain, language seems to crumble or collapse, that its vocabulary dwindles and perhaps stops short at the encounter with this intensity. It is also accurate that extreme pain seems to endanger our very humanity as we cry and scream, paying no heed to how we treat or speak to others around us. In addition, it is reasonable to argue that pain is perhaps the most direct and fierce experience we have of our utter withdrawal from others. On the one hand, when pain overwhelms us, we feel it with all its force and totality so that we very soon become our pain; on the other hand, we are completely helpless when trying to put it into words, describe it, or communicate it to others. These discordances serve, in many senses, as the basis of the firm grip pain has as a unique paradigm among the array of other internal states and feelings, which are all, no doubt, private and inaccessible, yet do not face us with such a degree of discrepancy.

When we reflect on the two aforementioned paradigms, as they take apart pain into its destructive and isolating components, it is important to bear in mind that the understanding of pain these two paradigms yield is not the mere joint product of each trait separately but also suggests something about an inseparability between them. For it is due to its fiercely destructive effect on our bodies as well as our language that pain isolates us, leaving us encapsulated in its a-linguistic, solipsistic realm. The two paradigms not only originate in the experience of pain, but they also fuel one another: there is no isolation without destruction, and vice versa. Moreover, this interdependency between the paradigms of pain is established via pain's relations with language. In other words, any account of pain as destructive or isolating, even when it does not explicitly discuss language, necessarily implies a strong and incontestable linguistic presence. This paradigmatic account of pain subsequently results in a resolute separation between language and the experience of pain.

We tend to adopt these binary accounts of pain, especially its negative traits, since they seem to correspond to our most natural intuitions regarding the experience of pain with which we are all so familiar (despite differences in context and intensity). This is why the two paradigms though abstract and theoretical, have such a powerful hold on us. But is the story so simple? Does our avoidance and fear of pain alone disclose its full essence? The challenge this book faces is to take serious account of our very basic, natural intuitions about pain, but at the same time, not to allow these intuitions to counterproductively narrow our perspective. The challenge is to retain this tension, since it touches on one of pain's crucial characteristics.

It is my argument that the bifurcation and antagonism between pain and language is rooted in the fact that the two theoretical paradigms fail to encompass the multifarious, complex nature of the experience of pain. In the theories constructed on the basis of these paradigmatic characterizations, pain can either be the essence of humanity or its abyss, either separating us from others or our direct connection to them; and finally, pain in these theories can either go with or against language. It is for this reason that pain "has" to be portrayed as humanity's most ferocious antithesis and a state that fundamentally threatens everything humanity stands for. It should already be clear, however, that the distinctive nature of pain can hardly be exhausted or done justice to by the impossibilities it harbors.

Let me point out some of the difficulties inherent to these paradigmatic views. First, while pain may leave us speechless, it also constitutes an insistent urge to express. In contrast to other internal or emotional states, pain may obliterate our linguistic abilities but at the same time demands a language. Pain drives us to express it and then demands to be heard and received by another (this demand is, clearly, not conditioned by the contingent question of whether it can or cannot be in fact received). It is therefore specifically in pain, more than in happiness or anger, for example, that we feel the depth of the implications of the discrepancy between the intensity of the feeling and the disintegration of our language. Being in a state of intense pain, hence, reveals itself to be inseparable from the compelling need to express it. Silent, mute pain is almost inconceivable.[38]

Second, pain does not merely deprive us of our humanity; it is also our vulnerability to pain that makes us human in the first place, that pins our humanity down, so to speak. We cannot fully experience the world and our existence in it without having some level of sensitivity to pain. Finally, while the experience of pain might mark a boundary between our feeling of ourselves and the feeling of others, it is at the same time the most direct and immediate manner by which we connect with other human beings (who all share this vulnerability to pain, regardless of linguistic or cultural differences). It is the pit from whose depths alone we can directly connect with other human beings, by empathizing or identifying. Pain encloses us in a hermetically solipsistic sphere, and yet it has an equal power to completely open us up to the possibility of sharing, participating, and reciprocating our pains with others.[39]

Moreover, if we consider the experience of pain solely from the perspective of those suffering it, we may be left with broken words and the collapse of our communicative capabilities. But the problematics inherent to the encounter between pain and language extend beyond the sufferer's body or speech, pertaining equally to those who witness the suffering of others. We all, not only those in pain, bear responsibility for the inexpressibility of pain. Every broken cry calls upon us, demands something from us, and has the potential to move us. This is another one of pain's distinct attributes: even when not spoken clearly or accurately defined, even when cried or moaned with the faintest breath, pain permeates us, stakes a claim on us—not on those who suffer from it, but most of all, on those who do not.

The weakness of the theories and paradigms I have been criticizing here is that their conception of pain is one-sided, that they settle on its "violent," depriving, and impairing side, evading the multifarious face of the experience of pain. Pain is human as well as dehumanizing; it is expressive while it simultaneously undermines our abilities to use language; though it separates, it also forcefully unites. I do not call into question or sidestep the violent confrontation between pain and language—who would want to deny it? Nor do I wish to aggrandize pain and present it in an exclusively positive light. Rather, my analysis comes to preserve and do justice to pain's uniquely complex nature as well as the distinctiveness of its encounter with language.

Herder

Many moments in the history of philosophy treat the above paradigmatic binaries as a self-evident premise. The confrontation between pain and language is found, most notably, in philosophical accounts of the origin of language, not only marking the birth of language but also, more importantly, shaping its self-definition. The philosophical understanding of the term "origin" is diverse and has a long, rich history. It includes the conception of the point of origin in temporal terms as a moment of genesis (most notably in eighteenth-century thought), and its understanding as essence (especially in the twentieth century after the so-called linguistic turn). Over and beyond advancing two different meanings of origin, these two theoretical orientations also imply a divergent understanding of the structure and nature of language itself. Yet, in spite of these differences, one common characteristic of the problem remains: the moment in which human language defines itself (is "born," whether temporally or essentially) is also the moment when its entanglement with its mirror image—pain—is problematized, and this occurs in two ways: as an insuperable confrontation as well as, simultaneously, an intimate kinship. The question of the origin of language is located, therefore, at the very threshold between linguistic expression and the expression of pain.

Since the moment of origin is conceived as the critical point of separation between the immediacy of the emotional and bodily realm in the experience of pain and the mediacy of linguistic articulation, it is there that, in order for language to be born, it must be divorced (or divorce itself) from its perfect "other," namely, animal being, bodily sensations and merely inarticulate acoustic exclamations. Language can thus only be born when it overcomes the power of the coarse bodily sensations in its endeavor to silence that power by way of replacing it with a word. Origin is hence dependent on separation: it is either in language or in the body, either man or animal. Language is born as it suppresses pain, out of pain, or rather, as it remains deeply entangled with pain—in each case the question of origin, far from implying a simple genesis or inception, presents us with the pangs of language.

With this conceptual framework in mind, there is one figure who stands out in the long line of thinkers who have discussed the origin of language: Johann Gottfried Herder (1744–1803). Herder was a man of his time insofar as his preoccupation with the origin of language is concerned. Like many of his contemporaries, he was interested with the philosophical possibility of narratives of origin (of society, language, etc.) and with their important implications for our understanding of language but also of the very essence and self-definition of the human (a coupling typical of eighteenth-century thought). Nevertheless, Herder stands out. He does not follow the prevalent conceptions of his time, especially not those separating bodily sensations and linguistic expression, or the idea that the body and its sensations have to be overcome, even surrendered, in order for language to emerge. Nor does he concur with the postulation of an unbridgeable gap between internal (emotion, sensation, feeling) and external linguistic expression. Instead, Herder understands language, first and foremost—that is, originally—to be intertwined with the suffering, pained, crying body, not separate from it.

These ideas are found most prominently in Herder's *Treatise on the Origin of Language* (1772).[40] Since this text is the very nucleus of the present book (and discussed in great detail in its first two chapters), I here offer only some preliminary remarks regarding its main drift and its importance for the argument in the book. The beginning of the *Treatise* encapsulate the crux of Herder's radical conception of language: "*Already as an animal, the human being has language*," he writes in the first line, and then continues: "All violent sensations of his body, and the most violent of the violent, the painful ones, and all strong passions of his soul immediately express themselves in cries, in sounds, in wild, unarticulated noises" (*Treatise* 65/*AS* 697). I elaborate on these lines extensively in chapter 2 but for now, let me just point at several crucial elements that immediately stand out: Herder situates the origin of language not in the merely human context but rather as pertaining to both man and animal. Moreover, the language at stake is also not exclusively human. In other words, the essence or origin of language is not limited to the human realm. Language does not define the human, crowning a linguistic lord of nature against the dark background of the animal but constitutes the origin of both. Second, for Herder, original linguistic expression is not articulate or propositional in any way and has nothing to do with communication. Third, primary linguistic expression is immediate and does not mediate; it is not conceptual but somatic; and notably, original linguistic expression is undifferentiated from the expression of pain.

Importantly, Herder does not posit this scene of a primordial creaturely existence of shared pains and cries as a prelinguistic stage of a primitive existence that occurred before the speaking human being emerged. Quite the contrary: for Herder there is no pre- to language, no world or being before, or without, language. His moment of "origin" belongs, therefore, not only to his unique understanding of language but also to a very specific conception that is much closer to essence than to a specific mythical moment in time (as we find in Condillac's story of the two children on a desert island who invent their own paradisiac, first language). In this sense, Herder's thought is much closer to twentieth-century philosophy (Wittgenstein, to take the most conspicuous example) than to his own time.[41]

This characterization of the origin of language has important implications where the "problem of other minds" is concerned. Instead of violently creating an unbridgeable rift between those in pain and the others around them, for Herder, pain's immediate expression in the cry is anything but private. Rather than distancing the onlookers, it touches them directly. The cry of "the language of sensations" in Herder's *Treatise* speaks to the whole of nature, and, more important than anything, receives an immediate response in a distinct form of sympathy. Pain does not separate: the sufferer is cut off neither from his or her ability to express nor from the sympathy of others. In the language of the two paradigms, no destruction, no isolation.

The uniqueness of Herder's theory lies in his almost unprecedented somatic conception of language. The *Treatise* presents an important moment from, and through, which we can rethink the binaries put forth by the two paradigmatic views detailed above. Instead of a violent antagonism, a dialectics emerges, between human and animal, body and language, isolation and communication. Herder's complex thought takes serious account of the body while he considers language, and of language in his attempt to grasp the body—human and animal alike—and its extreme sensations, specifically pain. The inseparability of language and sensation that forms the heart of Herder's theory of language is by no means trivial in the philosophical accounts of language of his time.

Pain's predominance in Herder's theory of the origin of language is present not only as a central theme or argument in the text. It appears already in the second line of the *Treatise*, with the introduction of the figure of the Greek hero Philoctetes. Herder mentions Philoctetes as part of his discussion of the original linguistic space occupied by the noncommunicative and direct expression of violent sensations. Here he refers to Philoctetes' wounding and the terrible pain it engendered: "A suffering animal, as much as the hero Philoctetes," writes Herder, "when overcome with pain, will whine!, will groan!, even if it were abandoned, on a desolate island, without the sight, the trace, or the hope of a helpful fellow creature" (*Treatise* 65/*AS* 697). In this single line, in one stroke, Herder presents almost all the threads underlying his theory of language: the relationship between human, animal, pain and language, communication or the absence thereof, and vocal expression.

Here in the *Treatise* Herder refers to Philoctetes only briefly, but his appearance is not accidental. Herder was preoccupied with this figure throughout his writings, not only in the context of language but also in his writings on aesthetics where he gives an elaborate account of Sophocles' drama and the problem of the interconnections between pain, expression, and sympathy (Sophocles, Herder writes, provided us with more psychology and knowledge of the human being than any philosopher could ever give).[42] In this present book, Herder's fascination with Philoctetes serves as an important axis with reference to which the relationship between pain and language, taken outside the boundaries of the two paradigms—destruction and isolation—can be reexamined.

Philoctetes

Philoctetes' story has been recounted in many versions beginning from antiquity, and it is still being staged and discussed today. Philoctetes appears in Homer's *Iliad*, Ovid's *Metamorphoses*, Apollodorus' *Epitome*, and Aristotle's *On Marvelous Things Heard*, to name just a few. The story was also rendered in numerous theatrical adaptations, including Aeschylus (457 BC) and Euripides (431 BC)—two versions that did not survive— Sophocles' famous version (409 BC), and other modern renderings by Jean-Baptiste Vivien de Chateaubrun (1755), André Gide (1898), Oscar Mandel (1961), Seamus Heaney (1961), Heiner Müller (1965), and even a brief appearance in Disney's 1997 *Hercules* (here Philoctetes is renamed "Phil").[43]

But Philoctetes' story is most famously told by Sophocles.[44] Let me recount the plot briefly.[45] Philoctetes was a Greek hero famous for his bravery and for his magic bow which never missed its mark, a bow given to him by Heracles before his death. The story begins when Philoctetes sails to Troy together with Odysseus, Agamemnon, Menelaus, and their soldiers. On their way, they stop at the island of Chryse to sacrifice an offering to the Gods. As they approach the holy place, they see a snake lying at the foot of the shrine. Philoctetes volunteers to approach it first and is bitten in his foot by the snake. Appearing insignificant at first, the snake bite turns into an infected wound. Philoctetes suffers terrible pain and begins to curse and scream out loud; his cries are horrific. The festering wound produces a horrible smell. Philoctetes' companions cannot stand the view of the wound and its smell. And above all they cannot bear Philoctetes' screams, which also prevent them from performing the religious ritual of sacrifice. They sail off to Lemnos, a close-by island, leaving behind the wounded, suffering Philoctetes. Philoctetes remains alone on the island for the next ten years, in the sole company of the local animals and with occasional brief visits from travelers who are passing through.

During this time, Philoctetes' wound neither heals nor gets better and he suffers continuously from terrible pain. According to the post-Homeric *Little Iliad*, Odysseus received a prophecy from Helenus according to which the only way for Greece to win the war against Troy was with the help of Heracles' magic bow, which was in the possession of Philoctetes. Odysseus decides to sail to Lemnos and get hold of the bow. However, concerned that Philoctetes will recognize him as one of the men who abandoned him on the desert island and refuse to forgive him, he takes along a young man, Neoptolemus, son of Achilles, to help him. Sophocles' play begins when the two men arrive at the island on which Philoctetes was deserted ten years earlier. Odysseus then offers Neoptolemus a concise, almost cold report of the events leading to Philoctetes' abandonment on the island, giving almost no account of Philoctetes' suffering. He then sends the young man in search of Philoctetes ordering him to cheat, lie, and do whatever is needed to obtain the bow. When Neoptolemus and Philoctetes first meet, Philoctetes tells his version of the story, which is of course wholly different from the one told by Odysseus. He recounts the circumstances of his injury and his terrible pain, but rather than his physical suffering he dwells on the unbearable pain of his abandonment. It is at this point that we begin to comprehend the proportions of the inhumanity of leaving Philoctetes alone on the island for ten long years. The physical disaster recedes into the background compared to the lack of compassion of Philoctetes' soldiers when they chose to sail away. Philoctetes was one of their own, a hero who did not deserve the punishment he suffered. Philoctetes remained alone in the solipsistic confines of this terrible pain, and the only answer to his cries of agony was their own echo resounding on the empty island.

The main question at this point of the story is whether Neoptolemus will stick to his commander's order and use every possible means to cheat Philoctetes out of his bow, or, having heard the latter's side of the events, will change his mind and tell Philoctetes the truth about the real purpose of his and Odysseus' journey to the island. The third act introduces precisely this ambivalence. The act begins after Neoptolemus has promised Philoctetes that he will rescue him from the island, but since at this stage the young man is still completely loyal to Odysseus, it is clear to us that he is lying to Philoctetes. Then, however, something happens. Philoctetes is suddenly struck by intense pain and freezes. During this pain attack, a dialogue develops between the two men: Neoptolemus, surprised by the sudden change in Philoctetes, keeps asking him what has happened, whereas Philoctetes, who is in such intense pain that he can hardly speak, replies with a series of exclamations—"A-a-a-a-h!" and "Ah, ah, ah, ah!"—that express his suffering. As Philoctetes passes out in pain, Neoptolemus undergoes a transformation: he decides to no longer obey Odysseus; he realizes that he is devoted to Philoctetes and eventually, to what he takes to be a true moral stance in the face of wrongdoing and suffering. He then confesses the truth to Philoctetes and offers to rescue him, this time sincerely. This is followed by a confrontation between the two and Odysseus (who finds them because he has been looking for Neoptolemus). Finally, Odysseus agrees to rescue Philoctetes, but the latter, resentful, now refuses to leave his desert island. The play ends with Heracles' invocation from heavens, convincing Philoctetes (who is enraged with Odysseus) to agree to be rescued from the island.

All versions of the story begin more or less similarly with the arrival of Odysseus (or Ulysses, his Latin name, in Gide's version) and his companion(s) at the desert island, to be followed by diverse accounts of the events that led to Philoctetes' affliction and abandonment ten years earlier. There are substantial differences in the plot, protagonists, and endings. Sophocles emphasizes moral questions of justice, revenge, and sympathy, whereas Chateaubrun's version includes a female figure, Philoctetes' daughter Sophie, with whom Odysseus falls in love. Müller presents the story in a political framework, focusing on the conflict between individual and state, ending the play with Philoctetes' murder by Neoptolemus, whereas in Mandel's account, Philoctetes is not alone on the island but has a servant by the name of Medon, whom Odysseus kills in the course of the play (in the original story Medon was the commander who succeeded Philoctetes when he was left behind in Lemnos). There is yet another rendition of the story, especially relevant in the context of my argument: this is Herder's own version published posthumously under the title "Philoctetes: Scenes with Song [*Philoktetes: Scenen mit Gesang*]."[46] A letter from the Riga publisher Hartknoch to Herder suggests that the drama was set to music by Johann Christoph Friedrich Bach around 1775, but Bach's music, or any evidence of its having been performed, did not survive.[47] In Herder's recasting of the story, Odysseus is absent and, as Weissberg points out, the focus is entirely on the relationship and dialogue between Philoctetes and Neoptolemus. In contrast to Sophocles, however, Herder focuses on neither Neoptolemus nor his tormenting conflict between the interest of the state and his commitment to Odysseus, nor again his own sympathy toward Philoctetes. Instead, it is Philoctetes who takes center stage, with a strong emphasis on his suffering and his inability to forgive, which deny him his rescue and eventual cure.[48]

Despite these divergences, however, what all accounts share is the postulate that Philoctetes is not a man "in" pain or one who "feels" pain. Pain has become Philoctetes' very identity: *he is his pain*.[49] Although Philoctetes obviously suffers, and it is so bad that he asks Neoptolemus to kill him (or in other versions, for instance Müller's, to cut off his foot),[50] nowhere is this pain depicted as not his own, as extraneous to him or foreign. During his solitary years it has become inseparable from him.[51] Philoctetes' wound has, indeed, a paramount presence in the plot as well as on stage, almost as if it were another character in the play. There is yet another aspect in the characterization of Philoctetes that is important to Herder and which explains his decision to allude to Philoctetes specifically in his text on the origin of language. Philoctetes is not only unique due to the terrible pain he suffers; he is also distinguished by how he expresses his pain. The intensity of his pain does not allow Philoctetes to speak; it robs him of his communicative abilities. But most of all, this pain is communicated in cries, groans, and screams, as if nevertheless insisting to be present to the ear: it is vocally expressed. This is the crux of Herder's fascination with Philoctetes: he is a speaking, civilized human being (that is, not prelinguistic in any way) yet, at the same time, a mere suffering body, immediately and instinctively crying out his pain. In other words, these two states, two modes of expression—one preeminently human, the other shared with the animals—are not mutually exclusive but exist concomitantly at one and the same time.

Language Pangs

Herder and Philoctetes make two appearances in this book: first, I discuss them in their respective historical frames of reference; the second time, I consider them as they reemerge in later philosophical texts, as genealogical echoes. I discuss Herder first in the context of eighteenth-century philosophy, against the background of the period's preoccupation with the problem of the origin of language, and in relation to figures such as Rousseau, writing about similar issues at the same time as Herder. However, almost two hundred years after the *Treatise,* Herder reappears as a central figure in a seminar Martin Heidegger taught in 1939. This reappearance suggests something of the importance of his ideas about pain, language, and expression; over and beyond featuring as a unique philosophical approach in his own time, he articulated ideas that resonate in the thought of one of the great philosophical minds of the twentieth century. Although Heidegger is mostly critical of Herder in his seminar, it is at the same time clear that Herder's ideas about language, pain, and chiefly, the importance of hearing, provide the foundation of some of Heidegger's later ideas.

Insofar as Philoctetes is concerned, his figure powerfully manifests how our thinking about pain is not limited to the event that caused it or the circumstances of its potential cure. Pain, as it is revealed in the story of Philoctetes, is not some external event but rather comes to constitute the entirety of his existence and innermost essence. When Philoctetes appears many centuries later in Herder's work, it is not only to illustrate the nature of pain and its dire consequences but as an epitome of the correspondence between pain and language and their entanglement. Furthermore, in an even more intricate configuration, the implications of the encounter between Herder and Philoctetes, which form the heart of this book's argument, lead me to yet another philosophical thinker of the twentieth century, namely, Stanley Cavell. Although Cavell discusses neither Herder nor Philoctetes explicitly, his ideas about pain, the challenge he poses to the problem of other minds, and his introduction and elaboration of the notion of "acknowledgment," offer a thought-provoking lever for my reexamination of the encounter between pain and language, especially because he addresses and overcomes the same binaries so central in my argumentation.

Some words about the book's structure and the following chapters. In chapter 2, I present in detail the two main texts in which Herder discusses Philoctetes. The first is the *Treatise* (1772) in which Herder presents his theory on the origin of language, a theory that is distinctly somatic: language arises from the depth of pain and is expressed in the crying voice. In this chapter I elaborate on the figure of Philoctetes who largely epitomizes Herder's understanding of language, including discussions of pain, the human-animal relation, sympathy, and expression. The second focus of chapter 2 is Herder's *Critical Forests* (1769), in which Philoctetes is not only briefly mentioned, as he is in the *Treatise*, but takes the foreground. Here, in the context of his criticism of Lessing, Herder considers the problem of sympathy and the expression of pain in Sophocles' *Philoctetes*. I read both texts from the perspective of three main terms: the cry of pain, silence, and sympathy.

Chapter 3 continues the discussion of the origin of language, moving from the language of sensations shared by humans and animals to what Herder presents as distinctly human language. Although Herder explicitly presents human language as what has separated itself from the immediacy of the expression of sensations, I argue that his statement here should be taken with a grain of salt. Notwithstanding the fact that human language is articulate and mediate, Herder keeps it very close to the fundamental principles of the language of sensations, especially where it comes to the emphatically acoustic dimension of both languages. If the language of sensations was founded on the production of sound in the form of a cry or groan, human language is all about hearing. With a radical shift from the customary conception of language rooted in speech and communication, Herder argues that it evolves from man's ability to listen—however, not to other human beings but rather to the natural world surrounding him. Herder uses the sense of hearing to establish a uniquely human linguistic orientation in the world, an idea that I develop in comparison to a related argument in Rousseau's theory of the origin of language.

In chapter 4 I follow ideas concerning sound and hearing, this time by way of a close reading of Heidegger's "On the Essence of Language: The Metaphysics of Language and the Essencing of the Word" (1939), a seminar on Herder's *Treatise*. From Heidegger's obscure preparatory notes to the seminar (as well as some of his students' notes), I reconstruct his interpretation of Herder, focusing on the sense of hearing and its importance to language. In this chapter, I point out what I take to be Herder's profound influence on Heidegger's later ideas—something that has been rarely noticed in the literature. Apart from the sense of hearing, another important topic in this chapter is the relationship between the internal and external, a question that often arises in the context of pain and its expression (do my "external" expressions, in cries or words, represent my "internal" feeling, etc.). Following Herder, Heidegger shows us that this is not the right question to ask, focusing instead on what he calls "the crossing-over," a unique space between inside and outside, sounds and silence. This is the space in which, according to Heidegger, language and hearing reside.

Chapter 5 returns to the presence of Philoctetes in Herder's thought and offers a thorough discussion of what I take to be the most important and suggestive scene in Sophocles' play: Philoctetes' pain attack. In this chapter I read this scene closely, gleaning from it some of Herder's central ideas about language, body, and language. My interpretation of the scene focuses on Philoctetes' cries of pain and how they constitute, rather than shatter, the possibility of sympathy for the pain of the other, which is the crux of the "problem of other minds." The problem of the possibility, or impossibility, of sympathy (already discussed in chapter 2), conjures yet another important figure in my discussion: Stanley Cavell. I turn to Cavell as a philosopher who brings the problem of pain together with that of language and sympathy, using the implications of skepticism to put forth his own approach to the possibility, or impossibility, of knowing the other's pain. In his "Knowing and Acknowledging," Cavell questions the obstinate epistemological inclination of the philosophical discussion about pain and instead suggests we think about our relationship to the pain of others not in terms of knowledge but rather of acknowledgment.

I then proceed to another version of the story, very unlike the previously mentioned ones, this time in André Gide's rendition: "Philoctetes; or the Treatise on Three Ethics" (1898). Gide presents Philoctetes as an altogether different figure: the ten solitary years on the island have not turned him into an angry, resentful man, but quite the opposite. In this version, Philoctetes, cast out on the island with no one to whom he can communicate his pain, has gradually rediscovered the expanse of language. Pain has not turned his language into a series of beastly, blunt cries but has rather taught him something about the beauty of language, a quality that only emerges when it is not used to communicate or refer to objects external to it. The language of Gide's Philoctetes is a poetic, free, and independent language, in which pain is no longer language's object of reference.

In the final chapter I tie the threads together as I return to pain, this time not as destructive and isolating, distinguished by the violence it exercises on language and on the possibility to think itself and the relation to the other concomitantly. Here pain appears as the condition of possibility not for language's demise but for its inception.

2

A Language of Pain

Herder and the Origin of Language

The Question of the Origin of Language

One of the first things one notices about Herder's "Treatise on the Origin of Language" (1772) is the abundant presence of oppositions in the text. This is evident, first, in the division of the *Treatise* into two parts, each treating one half of the Berlin Academy's prize-essay question. The first part asks: "Supposing men abandoned to their natural faculties, are they in a position to invent language?" (*Treatise* 65–127/*AS* 697–767); the second asks: "And by what means will they arrive at this invention?" (*Treatise* 127–164/*AS* 769–810). The split is to be viewed, however, as not merely formal, but rather, as a principle governing Herder's entire view of language. He begins the *Treatise* with a detailed description of the language of sensations (*eine Sprache der Empfindung*), which he describes as an immediate law of nature (*die unmittelbares Naturgesetz*), an original language (and not pre-language) man shares with animals. But then, only nine pages later, he expresses his astonishment that "philosophers, that is, people who seek distinct concepts, were ever able to arrive at the idea of explaining the origin of human language from this cry of the sensations. For is human language not obviously something completely different?" (*Treatise* 74/*AS* 708). Herder adds that since the only linguistic creatures we know are human beings, there is no sense in beginning our investigation of language elsewhere, or more securely, other than "with experiences concerning the difference between animals and human beings" (*Treatise* 77/*AS* 711). Herder uses similar statements in criticizing some of his contemporaries' approaches to the problem of the origin of language, for instance, referring critically to Rousseau, whose intelligence "was for a moment able to make it [language] arise from that source [of sensation]" (*Treatise* 76/*AS* 710), or elsewhere alluding to Maupertius' failure to "separate the origin of language sufficiently from these animal sounds" (*Treatise* 77/*AS* 710–711).[1] Herder grounds the breach between the two languages by way of the clear separation between human and animal: animal language amounts to an instinctive, immediate expression of violent passions and sensations, whereas human language is a reflective, mediated way of taking awareness; animals express themselves in cries and groans, whereas humans produce signs and words.

Herder thus questions the possibility that human language, the human mind's supreme analytical instrument, be thought of as a continuation of, or even in association with, the primary language of unconscious primordial sensations, and he adopts a stance that seems, initially, to be very close to that of the Enlightenment. It would accordingly be impossible to trace a continuous path from an expressive language common to human and animal to a referential, representative apparatus associated exclusively with humans, and implausible to move from immediacy to reflective awareness.[2] Herder consequently formulates what he conceives to be the superior status of human over animal language, with the former being a reflective apparatus used for communication and abstract thought and the latter used solely for the immediate expression of instincts. Rather than a quantitative progression, Herder assumes a qualitative leap between the two languages. From his perspective, since the human capacity of understanding cannot be added as some external supplement to the animal, a cry can accordingly never be organized into language, cannot simply develop into language.[3]

This initial dissonance is probably the reason that many interpreters of Herder's theory of language begin their analysis not at the beginning of the *Treatise* but rather from its second section, which explicitly considers human, reflective language.[4] While there is no doubt that the *Treatise* is mainly devoted to human language and its difference from animal forms of expression (only nine pages out of about a hundred are devoted to the language of sensation), Herder nevertheless chooses to begin the text with a description of this different language, the original language of nature and its living creatures, of which man is only one species. This choice is not accidental.

Before I begin with a close reading of the *Treatise*, it is worthwhile to glance at Herder's "Fragments on Recent German Literature" written only three years before the *Treatise*, where he presents some instructive insights about the problem of origin (*Ursprung*).[5] In *Fragments* Herder describes the quest for origins as a sweet dream of attaining some all-encompassing knowledge, a dream that remains essentially unsatisfied, as it continually generates further questions: "Was it always that way? How did it become? In the end therefore this yearning has strayed in its ascent up to that bold summit on which it appears like a cloud-creature: that of wanting to know the origin itself, of either experiencing it historically or explaining it philosophically or guessing it poetically" (*Fragments* 52). The yearning for knowledge has become, in Herder's words, a "cloud creature" or has gone astray, since the dream of the possibility of identifying a true, pure point of origin, at the same time generates the problematic desire to *really* experience or explain it, that is, to reconstruct it qua origin, as it really was.

In immersing ourselves solely in the search for origins, Herder claims, we tend to create a fissure between the moment of origin and the existing state of affairs, thus running the risk of missing (*entgehen*) an important part of the history of the case at hand. Language, to take his prominent example, grows and develops out of its origin just "like the tree from its root. . . . In the seed lies the plant with its parts, in the spermatozoon the creature with all its limbs, and in the origin of a phenomenon the whole treasure of elucidation through which the explanation of the phenomenon becomes *genetic*" (*Fragments* 53). Herder's genetic explanation (which he began to conceive here but later developed into a more detailed and established method in his philosophy of history) foregrounds an important part of his claim: an origin is never entirely separate (temporally or otherwise) from the phenomenon that developed out of it, therefore, when following our "sweet dream" of origin we should never search for it too far. Any phenomenon, not least language, is imbued with its original elements, which, even if invisible or buried, reside in its every constituent.

According to Herder, people have explained the origin of language as a divine gift to humans (this is Süßmilch's position, which Herder criticizes in several places); they have situated it in the speech organs (as though these are enough, even if found in an ape); sought it in animal vocalizations of passion; looked for it in the imitation of nature's sounds; and finally, sought it in mere convention and agreement, that is, in sociality: "These so numerous, unbearable falsehoods which have been stated about the human origin of language have in the end made the opposite opinion almost universal. But I hope that it will not remain so" (*Treatise* 90/*AS* 724–725). For Herder, the origin of human language can be accounted for only when taking the human being as the crux of the argument, and can never be sought in any external cause (animal, society, or divine origin). It seems then, that Herder is explicitly, even fervently, defending the binaries governing the *Treatise*, to the point of suggesting that without them, no origin of language can be accurately explained.

Returning to the problem of the connection between the original language of sensation and human language by way of putting the two texts—*Treatise* and *Fragments*—side by side, it becomes clear that Herder speaks in a dual voice. On the one hand, he advocates a genetic view, to the effect that we must think the two languages together; on the other hand, he explicitly differentiates between the language of sensation and human language, explicitly arguing for the philosophical importance of their separation. However, more than being a text about the essence of human language, the *Treatise* profoundly wrestles with the problem of origin (*Ursprung*), and it is therefore important that we begin our investigation at its very beginning. I propose that despite Herder's undeniable and explicit claims regarding the contradiction between the two languages, we set aside his assertions for now and carefully excavate the distinct dialectical correspondence between the two languages in the *Treatise*, a correspondence that, as I will show in detail, Herder's text in fact constitutes. This is not achieved easily with a philosopher like Herder, whose texts are filled with inner contradictions and a manifold of not-always consistent versions of similar ideas. That said, the force of Herder's philosophy is revealed precisely when we learn to treat these inconsistencies as productive rather than indicating a weakness in his arguments. I begin, then, with a reading that might at first seem to go against Herder's own arguments but is soon revealed to be loyal to his conception of language in the *Treatise*. Let us, then, take the text's very beginning seriously and pay attention to our own hesitation regarding Herder's self-reservations.

Pain and the cries of pain do not open the *Treatise* merely in order to disappear. Or perhaps one might argue that their disappearance, no sooner than they emerged, is in itself crucial for Herder and for our understanding of his argument. Being in pain and vigorously expressing it is part of being human and of having a language, even if these cries are subdued or smothered as human language develops away from the original language of sensation. Herder's renowned theory of reflective human language[6] is therefore to be understood neither as a mere advanced stage of original language nor, clearly, as its negation. The beginning of the *Treatise* is crucial precisely because it provides a painstaking account of the *other* of human language, that which is never completely abolished and always finds its way into the most articulate, conceptual, and abstract linguistic expressions. This casts an interesting light on why Herder does not endorse the claim for a divine origin of human language (as his rival Süßmilch does) but establishes instead an inherent connection between human and animal language.[7] It is specifically this kinship (rather than that between the human and the divine) that allows him to establish the strong connection between language and pain and the passions. A divine origin can emphasize human sovereignty over the natural world or the supremacy of reason, but it is incapable of pointing at pain and passion as the nucleus of language. Human language is "already" (*schon*), to use Herder's formulation, there from the very beginning.

Herder's Two Figures of Philoctetes

The *Treatise* opens with a compelling description of a primordial language consisting of forceful and immediate expressions of powerful sensations;

however, although Herder designates this language as animalistic in nature, he chooses to introduce the human figure of Philoctetes at its very beginning. Philoctetes is mentioned on the first page of the *Treatise*, almost in passing, when Herder describes a suffering animal's cry of pain and compares it to that of Philoctetes, abandoned on the desert island (*Treatise* 65/*AS* 697).[8] Philoctetes is presented here as producing a primordial, natural howl of pain which for Herder exemplifies something of the original language shared by humans and animals, a language he designates as the "language of sensation" (*Sprache der Empfindung*). The appearance of cries of pain as the background to a systematic, all-encompassing theory of human language has a fundamentally evasive effect whose implications are more telling than they may seem at first. Philoctetes' presence at the beginning of the *Treatise* is similarly elusive. At first a trifling, even accidental, example, Philoctetes' oblique presence has substantial implications, not only for the overall appreciation of Herder's complex relationship to the figure of Philoctetes, but foremost, for a rigorous evaluation of his theory of language. The importance of Philoctetes lies, I argue, in the manifest challenge he poses to Herder's ostensibly strict separation between the animal and human, immediate physical, and reflective human expression, and finally, between the original language of sensation and the human, reflective one.

Philoctetes' appearance in the *Treatise* is, however, not Herder's first allusion to the figure in his oeuvre. In 1769, the same year in which the Berlin academy announced its prize-essay question on the origin of language, Herder published "Critical Forests" (anonymously), a text whose first part presents a detailed discussion of Sophocles' theatrical representation of Philoctetes.[9] The source of Herder's fascination with this figure is a story about another suffering hero, namely, Laocoön, the Trojan priest who, together with his two sons, was strangled by two giant serpents the gods (Athena in one version, Poseidon in another) sent to punish him. The story of Laocoön and the aesthetic representations of his terrible suffering were discussed by Johann Joachim Winckelmann (1755), whose interpretation was later famously criticized by Gotthold Ephraim Lessing (1766).[10] The context of Winckelmann's and Lessing's discussion is the question of the relationship between the visual arts (especially sculpture) and poetry—a common concern of eighteenth-century aesthetics. Both discuss a Greek marble sculpture (or "group") representing Laocoön and his sons struggling with the snakes and compare it with a passage from Virgil's *Aeneid*, describing the same scene.

Lessing's *Laocoön* drew Herder's attention immediately on its publication in 1766 and he claimed to have read it through three times in a single sitting.[11] Herder presents the results of his meticulous study of Winckelmann and Lessing in the first part of "Critical Forests" (or the "First Grove" as he calls it) under the title: "Dedicated to Mr. Lessing's Laocoön."[12] I return to *First Grove* in detail later in this chapter, but for now let me just indicate three important issues this text raises. First, the crux of Herder's debate with Lessing is the cry of pain and the problem of its aesthetic representation; second, Herder considers this problem in the context of the question of sympathy; third, he does not unfold his argument as part of the alternative interpretation of Laocoön but rather with a detailed account of another figure, namely, Philoctetes. Lessing discusses Philoctetes against the background of his central figure, Laocoön; Herder, by contrast, puts Philoctetes in the front, using Sophocles' version of his story as the basis of his claims.

Herder's reference to Philoctetes in the *Treatise* could be attributed to the author's intense preoccupation with this figure when he wrote *First Grove,* at an earlier time. We could say that Philoctetes' story was still at the back of his mind when he began to work on the *Treatise,* thus finding its way into the text as an example. I understand this differently. First, Philoctetes' figure remains central for Herder and appears once again two years after the *Treatise* in *Philoktetes: Scenen mit Gesang* (1774), Herder's own version of the story.[13] Second, I take the abridged reference to Philoctetes in the *Treatise* to function like an anchor thrown into the text from Herder's critical discussion of Lessing, thereby providing the link between Herder's aesthetic discussion of the figure and his account of language and its origins. Taking up this connection, however, turns out to require a more complicated move than the mere bringing together of Herder's aesthetics and linguistic theories. Although Philoctetes indeed appears in both texts with a similar emphasis on his terrible pain, Herder presents him in two entirely different, even contradictory, ways.

In the *Treatise,* Philoctetes is an instinctive, suffering, howling animal, whereas in *First Grove* he features as an admirable hero who endures his pain without allowing any instinctive, involuntary cries to escape. Did Herder change his mind about the figure? Or is he perhaps pointing at an essential, inner contradiction in Philoctetes' own character? In my reading, the crying and the silent Philoctetes are not as mutually exclusive as they might seem; in fact, they are inseparable and depend on one another. Deciphering the relationship between the two proves, moreover, to be essential for our understanding of Herder's conception of language and the role of pain plays in it. I begin with a close reading of the *Treatise* and *First Grove,* centering on Herder's two accounts of Philoctetes and his expressions of pain, and then propose they can be brought together into one consolidated figure which serves, I will argue, as an epitome of Herder's theory of language.[14]

The Crying Philoctetes: Herder's Theory of the Origin of Language

Herder begins his consideration of the origin of language with a description of a primordial, original language grounded in violent, passionate cries of pain. This "language of sensation" (*Sprache der Empfindung*), as Herder calls it, is not distinctly human but designates an expressive apparatus shared by human beings and animals alike. Such a beginning for a text on the origin of human language is significant, even striking. When the question of the origin of language is posed in the eighteenth century it usually refers to, or at least implies, the question of the origin of *man*. Any exploration of the invention of language by men "abandoned to their natural faculties," as the Berlin academy puts it, would mean tackling what it is that makes the human being human, what distinguishes him from the rest of nature and specifically from nonspeaking animals. Herder seems to undertake the problem from a surprising angle: instead of setting out with a discussion of the conditions for the constitution of a distinctively *human* language, he starts by putting humans together with animals, belonging in a communal natural world, sharing one and the same "language."

The *Treatise* opens with the following lines: "Already [Schon] as an animal, the human being has language. All violent [heftigen] sensations [Empfindungen] of his body, and the most violent of the violent, the painful ones, and all strong passions [starke Leidenschaften] of his soul immediately [unmittelbar] express themselves in cries, in sounds, in wild, unarticulated noises" (*Treatise* 65/*AS* 697).[15] This opening sentence enfolds several claims. First, the human being always had language. Hence there is no temporal moment of origin at work for Herder but rather a structure in which human beings, by their very being human, have always been linguistic creatures; put differently, what defines the human *as* human is his or her being linguistic. According to Peter Hanly, Herder's *Schon als Tier* means accordingly, that insofar as man is an animal, he has language.[16] This claim, however, has two conflicting meanings. On the one hand, the human being is not conceived as a speaking animal; that is, man is not an animal to whom language has been added, as if it were some extraneous component. On the other hand, sharing the primary language of sensation with the animal the human being is not defined by having a language. While the *Treatise* opens with a conceptual distinction between human and animal, the ground of this distinction is not immediately clear. This opening also implies that the human being was *once* an animal. Here humans *are* indeed constituted in time: *already* (Schon) when he was an animal, the human being possessed language.

In order to get a grip on the unique starting point of Herder's text, we need to carefully study the nature of a human-animal language that is original, not in the temporal sense but rather, original as in essential (I return to this point later on). Herder describes the original language as first and foremost expressive. It emanates from violent bodily sensations and the passions of the soul and is expressed immediately in screams and inarticulate nonverbal exclamations. The immediacy that Herder refers to here is of course not temporal in nature, suggesting that the cry follows the sensation in time, but rather, points at *unmittelbarkeit*: the opposite of a mediated, conceptual, or abstracted expression.

Herder stresses that these sounds produced by the "suffering animal" (animal here referring to beast as well as human) are not meant to transmit any designative or propositional linguistic content. These expressions of pain emerge as physical expressions of physical agonies. Herder, however, argues that these primordial natural sounds are language: "These groans, these sounds, are language. Hence there is a language of sensation [Sprache der Empfindung] which is an immediate law of nature" [unmittelbares Naturgesetz] (*Treatise* 66/*AS* 698). Herder could have labeled this a "prelinguistic" stage, or a "forerunner" of language, but instead he treats these violent nonverbal expressions as language per se. The reason for this, among other things, inheres in Herder's conception of language as an evolving entity with an inner movement that drives it forward rather than a static and discrete divine "gift" bestowed on human beings.

It is specifically and emphatically pain that Herder foregrounds here. What distinguishes pain from the other passions or sensations is not only its ferocity or intensity but also the nature of the connection between this violent sensation and its immediate expression. As I outlined in chapter 1, the cry of pain seems to be almost indistinguishable from the sensation of pain, so that when one cries out in pain, this cry is not a description or even designation of a sensation, but rather its immediate, direct expression. The choice of physical pain as the paradigmatic origin of language, therefore, appears to rest on two of pain's attributes: pain is, on the one hand, the tangible bodily affect par excellence; on the other, it is the feeling most patently expressed by the body in sounds and cries. Herder's claim regarding a language founded on pain offers a model of linguistic externalization that is fundamentally physical, an instinctual outpouring springing from the experience of pain. A parallel therefore exists between the feeling of *physical* affliction and its *physical* expression in language so that the body becomes the point where feeling and its expression intersect. I emphasize this so as to argue that Herder's choice of pain as an exemplary "violent sensation" is not only related to its vehemence or ability to transgress the boundaries between body and soul. It concerns the way in which pain and its distinct form of expression corresponds with Herder's understanding of human language as first and foremost *expressive* (rather than designative or propositional).

Herder focuses not so much on describing the intense, anguished experience of animal pain; instead, he concentrates on pain's unique mode of expression:

> A suffering animal . . . when overcome by pain, will whine!, will groan! . . . It is as though it breathed more freely by giving vent to its burning, frightened breath; It is as though it moaned away part of its pain, and at least drew into itself from the empty atmosphere new forces for getting over its pain, by filling the deaf winds with groaning. . . . *Here is a sensitive being* [empfindsames Wesen] *which can enclose none of its lively sensations within itself, which in the first moment of surprise, even without volition and intention, has to express* [äußern] *each of them in sound.* (*Treatise* 65–66/*AS* 697–698)

Language begins with pain; but the primordial link between pain and language is neither representation nor designation. Language's original sounds therefore, do not describe pain or refer to it: for Herder the sensation of pain is not language's object. Our primary and fundamental expressions are screams, howls, and animal groans, and the origin of language is plainly physical (the creature *äußert,* literally externalizes, the sounds of its pain); it springs from the violent confrontation between pain's overwhelming quality and language's correspondingly irrepressible vigor. Considering this against the background of my argument in chapter 1, Herder's description, we notice, is antithetical: language does not collapse in the face of pain; it is not revealed as weak and incompetent. On the contrary, the more vigorous the pain, the more forceful is its linguistic expression.[17]

Language's original cry issues forth when the body, physically speaking, cannot contain the pain, when pain becomes excessive and pours out in expression (*Ausdruck*), ex-pressed. The literal meaning of the German *Aus-druck* (out-press) is important here: the word signifies a pressing outward or expelling and literally designates how pain is emitted from the suffering body into the surrounding atmosphere. Pain is not spoken of, described, or pointed at; it is not translated into any form of propositional content or statement. It is simply and strongly let out, physically expressed, out of, away from the suffering body. Herder uses the creature's "breathing" to emphasize the physical, involuntary characteristics of this original cry: the breath of air physically externalizes, which in turn physically forces out some of the pain so as to relieve the body of its unbearable suffering. The correlation between breath and pain appears also in "On Cognition and Sensation of the Human Soul" written just a few years later (1778), where Herder contemplates the effects of breath on the living body: "In the case of a sick person, in the case of a groaning person, how inhaling gives courage, whereas each sigh so to speak breathes away forces." He then continues by quoting the Persian poet Sadi who writes that "a breath that one draws into oneself strengthens, a breath that one releases from oneself gives joy to life."[18] The immediate expression of pain is as natural as the rhythm of breathing for the living body. Pain is therefore almost unthinkable without its expression in sound.

Although constructing his discussion on the nature of pain, Herder argues that it is unimportant whether the expressed emotion is fear, pain, or passion. Expressive language does not focus on any specific determination; it draws attention to the general emotive picture, to which it only points but does not depict (*Treatise* 67/*AS* 699–700). We therefore have a "language of sensation." The choice of pain as exemplary allows Herder to demonstrate something important not only for the origin of linguistic expression but also regarding the unique connection between the sensation of pain and its cry. The case of pain's expression demonstrates most clearly that there is no question of mediation at the most fundamental level of linguistic expression: it immediately expresses an immediate sensation. The implications of Herder's claim touch on the crucial difference between immediate expression, on the one hand, and designative, communicative representation, on the other. This is also where the role of the figure of Philoctetes begins to become clear. I describe the story in detail in chapter 1, for now it is important to take note that the story revolves around two main issues: the experience of pain (Philoctetes' snake bite), and the problem of sympathy (the relationship between Philoctetes and Neoptolemus). Philoctetes epitomizes a man whose terrible pain has turned him into an animal (this is how most interpreters see it), and Neoptolemus represents a transformation from aloofness into all-encompassing sympathy. It is from these two poles that Herder invokes the figure of Philoctetes in the *Treatise*.

Philoctetes appears in the above quoted paragraph from Herder's *Treatise* as part of an analogy: "A suffering animal, *as much as* the hero Philoctetes, when overcome by pain, will whine!, will groan! even if it were abandoned, on a desolate island, without the sight, the trace, or the hope of a helpful fellow creature" (*Treatise* 65/*AS* 697), my emphasis). Herder treats Philoctetes as exemplary in his unique expressions of pain: the terrible animal-like cries, howls, and desperate screams that resonate for such a long time on his island.

The play's acoustic slant is evident from its very beginning. Odysseus is the first to recount the story of Philoctetes' abandonment, emphasizing his unbearable screams that filled the entire camp, which drove him and his soldiers away, compelling them to abandon Philoctetes.[19] In Müller's version of the play, Philoctetes himself describes his screams as marking the invisible boundaries of the inescapable expanse of his pain. He turns to Odysseus, trying to convey how it feels to be trapped in one's own pain. If I shall pierce your foot, Philoctetes says to him, you will begin crawling and running: "To no avail, running from your screams/To no avail, screaming louder as you run,/And louder in you if you stop your ears. . . . Have you learned to scream? (*Müller, Philoc.* 247). What is so compelling about Müller's version is that it is not pain itself that traps Philoctetes in his suffering body; it is, rather, the expressions of his pain in screams and cries that become his fateful snare (what Levinas describes as the "impossibility of nothingness").[20] Contra to Herder's description in the *Treatise* of the cry of pain as a relieving externalization of an excess of suffering, for Müller's Philoctetes the cry remains internal, so that any attempt to escape it would entail escaping one's very self. Philoctetes conveys the suffering inherent to pain to Odysseus not by having him imagine the physical sensation of the affliction or wound but by drawing him into the isolated "island" of its expression in sound.

Enclosed in his own isolated, speechless world, Philoctetes' long, solitary life on the desert island is revealed as a cruel metaphor: his isolated existence is not merely the result of his fellow soldiers' abandoning him but has to do more with the violent isolation pain decrees. Philoctetes is not only left alone on an island; he becomes an island himself.[21] This is the loneliness of being forsaken by his peers as well as the solitude his pain imposes, a loneliness he is faced with when the only possible response to his cry is an echo. When the chorus describes Philoctetes' suffering to Neoptolemus it sings: "And she whose mouth has no bar, Echo, appearing far off responds to his bitter cries of lamentation" (*Sophocles, Philoc.* 179–181). When Philoctetes is about to leave the island setting out for Troy, he bids farewell to Echo calling to the mountain that has "brought back to me a groan answering my voice as the storm assailed me!" (1455).[22] Echo is a unique embodiment of a combination between a purely acoustic entity and utmost passivity: its sound can only re-sound. If Echo was Philoctetes' only companion in his lonely years on the island, then obviously the only sounds he heard were his own, resonating the very fact of his loneliness. Pain, therefore, is neither a foreign agency attacking us from outside nor some kind of content stored away in our interiority, just waiting to be externalized and expressed. Both pain and its expression turn out to be nothing other than our very selves: sensation as well as expression.

The first appearance of Philoctetes in Sophocles' play is yet another demonstration of the importance of the sonic element. It is only after two hundred lines that Sophocles brings Philoctetes on the stage (until then his story was only told in third person), yet now too this initial appearance is through the sound he produces, the sound of pain. During the conversation between Neoptolemus and the chorus, Sophocles inserts a stage direction: "An offstage moan is heard" (*Sophocles, Philoc.* 200).[23] "A sound rang out!" sings the chorus, "such as might haunt the lips of a man in agony" (203–204). The chorus identifies Philoctetes by way of his moaning. They don't see, but *hear* him approaching: "There's no mistaking." But over and beyond being manifestations of Philoctetes' pain—these sounds are also the expression of suffering as such, the sound of suffering: "I know the sound of suffering" (206), Meineck and Woodruff translate.

It is only then, after he makes himself heard, that Philoctetes enters the stage, flesh and blood, wounded, and carrying his bow and arrows.[24]

The dominance of sound is, however, not only mediated through the portrayal of Philoctetes' agonizing vocal expressions but also appears in the context of hearing. The suffering of abandonment has one overwhelming implication: even where they are expressive and articulate, Philoctetes' cries cannot be heard by anyone. This is conveyed in the description of his first encounter with Neoptolemus. The chorus notices him approaching by the sound of his cries (see especially 201–208); and as soon as he, in turn, sees Neoptolemus he refers to the latter's voice. "O sound that I loved. O speech I have missed/So long," Philoctetes turns to Neoptolemus, "Long long I heard it solely from my mouth/When pain dug the cries out of my throat. Unfeeling rocks returned my cries to me. My ears crave another voice. Live then, live/Because you have a voice. Speak up, you Greek" (*Müller, Philoc.* 230).[25] After so many solitary years, it is the sound of the human voice that moves Philoctetes the most. What Neoptolemus actually says does not matter; he may lie and cheat or hurt with his words: but he speaks, he uses language. The animal is transformed into a human being not by way of expression but by way of hearing and recognizing the voice of another man.

As Liliane Weissberg points out, Herder's reference to Philoctetes is in fact an abbreviated version of a longer passage from an earlier draft of the *Treatise*.[26] In this earlier manuscript, Herder emphasizes the sonic constituent of Philoctetes' cries, which fill the whole of nature with an immediate expression in voice and language (*unmittelbare Stimme und Sprache*). Herder uses words such as *Klagetönen* and *Wehklagen* (plaintive sounds and lamentations), foregrounding the unique musicality of Philoctetes' animal-like shrieks; in the words of Sophocles' chorus: "The only answer to his hopeless cries/Is the perpetual call of Echo,/Far, far away in the distance" (*Sophocles, Philoc.* 183–190).[27] But this acoustic emphasis is also evident in Herder's own musical version of Philoctetes' story, "Philoctetes: Scenes with Song" [*Philoktetes: Scenen mit Gesang*] (1774). Both texts manifest the interruption of speech in the face of pain. Herder's *Philoctetes* is characterized by its emphasis on the sounds of pain. His stage directions read: "Die Töne hemmen, ändern sich, der Schmerz beginnt" [The sounds hamper, (they) change, the pain begins]. According to Weissberg, music introduces pain here by interrupting language, a *Hemmung*, that is expressed as internal to language, leaving a space for pain's appearance. In the drama, these interruptions are acoustic; in the *Treatise*, they are evinced visually, between the written characters on the page. "While Herder attempts to write about the cry," Weissberg writes, "its representation—an inadequate, but the only possible, one—strives to overcome the written letter, and tries to document the performance of the eruption and silencing of sounds. The text tries to stage, enact, the question of origin within its articulation."[28]

Scarry refers to Philoctetes when she describes the destructive, isolating facets of pain exemplified by the hero's solitude after being deserted on the island, a solitude of "absolute privacy with none of its safety, all the self-exposure of the utterly public with none of its possibility for camaraderie or shared experience."[29] This destructive solitude does not only take the form of the secluded place in which Philoctetes finds himself on waking up alone; Scarry describes it also in terms of pain's ability to reduce us to a "pre-language of cries and groans," regressing to a primitive nonhuman stage.[30] The destructive force of his pain has not only affected Philoctetes' body and world but also robbed him of his ability to use language in a social, communicative environment, thus turning him, in Sophocles' version, into a prelinguistic and therefore, prehuman creature. When Odysseus describes how Philoctetes cried and howled as he was wounded, he uses a vocabulary that is explicitly associated with savage, animal sounds (*Sophocles, Philoc.* 10); Philoctetes himself, describing his own agony, uses similar phrases begging Neoptolemus to not "shrink back in horror" at his "savage aspect" (ἀπηγριωμένον) (or in Meineck and Woodruff's translation: "I know, I must look like a wild man") (226–227).[31] Philoctetes' cave is correspondingly depicted as containing merely a bed of leaves and a piece of wood used as a cup—a distinctly animal form of existence, or at least, nonhuman. When Neoptolemus searches for him at the beginning of the play, he looks for his footprints as if he is tracking down an animal. This animal-being is expressed most emphatically during Philoctetes' pain attack when his speech literally crumbles into mere syllables and cries.

Let me suggest a different reading of Herder's reference to Philoctetes. Philoctetes appears in the *Treatise* not to portray a figure who, when in intense pain, regresses into a beast-like, primitive state. Herder accentuates a wholly different aspect of the story: Philoctetes is well aware that he is alone on the island, that no one can hear his cry, empathize with him, or help him in any way. He does not expect to be understood and helped, or even heard; that is to say, his language is essentially not communicative or propositional. It is important to bear in mind, nevertheless, that though animal-like in their instinctive immediacy, Philoctetes' groans and howls do not turn him into an animal. Philoctetes is not a beast but a human being subject to the most extreme and intense (physical and psychological) suffering, a condition in which his humanity does not clash with his animal nature but is rather subsumed by it. In Herder's linguistic theory, Philoctetes offers a figure that embodies the human as well as animal facet of being at one and the same time, so that the two cease being mutually exclusive properties. These two facets together burst forth with Philoctetes' appalling cry; this is the cry that drove away his fellow soldiers who abandoned him alone on the island, the same, agonizing cry that forms the crux of Lessing's text.

The Silent Philoctetes: Herder's Aesthetic Theory

In his study of the suffering Philoctetes in *First Grove*, Herder offers an entirely different analysis of his expression of pain. Here Philoctetes is not an instinctive animal giving direct expression to physical adversities but an honorable hero, who endures his unbearable suffering with impressive restraint. Herder's argument appears against the background of Winckelmann's and Lessing's accounts of Laocoön. The three authors—Winckelmann, Lessing, and Herder—can be perceived to intersect at one single point: that of the cry. The three texts at hand are all preoccupied with the cry of pain and its expression in the different aesthetic mediums. Each author interprets Laocoön's expressions of pain and explains the differences between sculpture and poetry, which are manifest in this context, in silence and cry. Although Herder writes the *First Grove* with deep admiration for Lessing—as is clearly manifest in his attentive close reading of Lessing's arguments—the text very soon delves into a fierce critique of the author who, according to Herder, "has gone astray" (*First Grove* 61).[32] To better understand Herder's account of Philoctetes in this text, we must briefly dwell on the debate between Lessing and Winckelmann that lies at the center of the former's famous *Laocoön*. Since it has been exhaustively studied, I shall not present this debate in detail but approach it from my own, specific angle, namely, Herder's concern with Philoctetes.[33]

Lessing launches *Laocoön* with a lengthy quote from Winckelmann's 1755 *Reflections*, where the latter compares Laocoön's and Philoctetes' expressions of pain: "Laocoön suffers, but he suffers like the Philoctetes of Sophocles; his anguish pierces our very soul, but at the same time we wish that we were able to endure our suffering as well as this great man does."[34] Contrary to Winckelmann, Lessing finds no similarity whatsoever between Laocoön's and Philoctetes' expressions of suffering and explains that whereas Laocoön nobly and quietly bears his pain, Philoctetes laments, cries, and fiercely curses using expressions that are anything but subdued or heroic.[35] Lessing stresses that Philoctetes' physical pain is not only unbearable to himself but that his impassioned, horrifying screams are also intolerable for his companions, causing them to abandon him on the desert island. Philoctetes in Sophocles' play is therefore characterized not only by his pain and its expression but also, and perhaps foremost, by his inability to kindle sympathy or pity in his companions' hearts. Lessing takes the occasion of his critique of Winckelmann's position to put forth his central argument in his book *Laocoön*, namely, that a clear boundary separates visual arts (mainly painting and sculpture), whose governing principle is spatial, and dramatic arts, regulated by temporal principles. Thus, his problem with Winckelmann's argument that Laocoön and Philoctetes suffer in the same way, rather than referring to any variance between the two men or their stories, involves the fact that each of the suffering heroes is depicted in a different aesthetic medium: Winckelmann's Laocoön is a statue, whereas his Philoctetes is a dramatic figure.

Since for Lessing, beauty is the supreme principle of visual arts, a sculptor cannot, by definition, strive for a faithful realistic representation of pain, as it would compromise the artwork's commitment to the law of beauty: "The demands of beauty could not be reconciled with the pain in all its disfiguring violence, so it had to be reduced. The scream had to be softened to a sigh, not because screaming betrays an ignoble soul, but because it distorts the features in a disgusting manner" (*Laocoön* 17). Lessing, however, develops and establishes his argument not only by way of a description of the different mediums and their artistic characterizations; he accentuates, rather, the way in which artistic representation affects its audience: "Simply imagine Laocoön's mouth forced wide open, and then judge! Imagine the screaming and look!" he writes, "From a form which inspired pity because it possessed beauty and pain at the same time, it has now become an ugly, repulsive figure from which we gladly turn away. For the sight of pain provokes distress; however, the distress should be transformed, through beauty, into the tender feeling of pity" (*Laocoön* 17). This is why Lessing is attracted to the sculptured Laocoön, a quiet, enduring figure, whose expressions of pain do not attack the viewers, so to speak, causing them to turn away, but rather allow them to stay close and develop a sense of sympathy and pity toward Laocoön's suffering.

Herder opens his *First Grove* with a replication of the opening of Lessing's Laocoön. Lessing quotes Winckelmann's "Laocoon suffers like the Philoctetes of Sophocles," and then asks: "But how does Philoctetes suffer?" Herder begins by what seems to be a continuation of the dialogue: "Let us open our Sophocles, let us read as if we were watching the drama," he writes. "Let the Philoctetes of Sophocles decide: how does he suffer?" (*First Grove* 55).[36] With this Herder opens a lengthy, detailed close reading and discussion of Lessing's arguments, taking them apart one by one into their smallest possible constituents. Instead of concentrating on Laocoön, however, he focuses on Sophocles' Philoctetes. In his subtle, albeit somewhat loose, account of Sophocles' version of the story, Herder presents a figure that not only diverges from Lessing's rendering, but also surprisingly contradicts his own earlier description of Philoctetes in the *Treatise*. Hence my claim regarding Herder's "two figures" or two versions of Philoctetes.

Instead of emphasizing Philoctetes' violent, animal-like cries of pain, in *First Grove* Herder accentuates the exact opposite: his admirably suppressed, heroic endurance of pain and its restrained expressions. Philoctetes does not cry out but enters the theatrical stage in "a sudden silence, in mute dismay . . . his face full of love, full of the self-restraint of the hero"; he "does not roar and rage . . . he whimpers. Nothing more? No, nothing more!" (*First Grove* 56). Herder's account of Philoctetes' silent endurance is a direct allusion to Winckelmann's account of the similarity between Laocoön's and Philoctetes' expressions of suffering:

> While suffering swells the muscles and contracts the nerves, the spirit armed with strength displays itself in the furrowed forehead,—the breast heaves with interrupted respiration, and with the suppression of the outbreak of feeling in his effort to contain and shut up the pain within himself. . . . The face is mournful, but there is no outcry. . . . Below the forehead, the struggle between pain and resistance is portrayed with the greatest wisdom; for while pain elevates the eyebrows, the effort to resist it presses the flesh just over the brows down upon the upper lid, so that the protruding brow almost covers it.[37]

Winckelmann presents Laocoön as a figure exemplifying "nature in extremity of suffering" together with the unmatched beauty of spiritual strength enabling the hero to admiringly subdue his suffering. This account becomes the ground for the transition Herder makes here from the discussion of Laocoön to that of Philoctetes.

Herder attributes this (as he believes) astounding description of Philoctetes' endurance to Sophocles, who

> has him do everything possible to prevent him from crying out—he raves, he groans, he pleads, he rages, breathlessly he comes to, and—passes out. What an agonizing scene! Perhaps the most intense expression ever demanded by a tragedy, which only a Greek actor could achieve. But what is the most intense form of expression in this agonizing scene, what is its keynote? A cry? Hardly, for Sophocles seems to take especial care to ensure that a cry is not the keynote. (*First Grove* 57)

For Herder, Sophocles' greatness lies in his ability to create a play that presents a scene of terrible suffering and pain without a single cry being uttered. Sophocles conjures a vast array of different degrees of anguish and their expressions (Herder calls this a *Gemälde des Schmerzes*, i.e., a painting or picture of pain),[38] which, taken as a whole, provide the spectator with "a picture of *subdued* and not *articulated* pain. . . . But the restraint, the agonized self-mastery, the long, silent struggles with his torment . . . are drawn out, they creep, and they are the keynote of the entire scene" (*First Grove* 57–58).

This is the heart of Herder's dispute with Lessing. Lessing discusses the nature of Philoctetes' pain and wound in detail so as to elucidate its inherent connection with the natural expression of the cry. Herder, on the other hand, seeks to concentrate on the theatrical nature of pain and therefore criticizes Lessing for putting his emphasis in the wrong place: "In that case," he writes, "I bid farewell to the theater! For I find myself in a hospital" (*First Grove* 76). Moreover, he adds, Philoctetes is so effective in moving the spectator to pity, not because he cries out his pain like animals do, but since he is able to contain it, endure it, in such a way that only a sigh, an "Ah!" escapes his mouth, a mere breath. Herder would agree with Lessing that Philoctetes is an emphatic representation of a man in pain; however, the audience experiences this pain all the more profoundly when its expression is withheld and not instinctively voiced out.[39]

We have, then, two very distinct accounts of Philoctetes in Herder. In the *Treatise,* Philoctetes is a "suffering animal" whose pain is immediately expressed in vigorous, primitive howls, a human who regresses to an animal state where language is nothing but a physical externalization of the sensation of pain. In *First Grove,* by contrast, we find an entirely different Philoctetes: a noble, strong hero who endures hellish suffering, both physical and mental, without letting his natural expressions pour forth. It is difficult to make sense of this inconsistency. These clashing figures of Philoctetes are even more striking if we bear in mind that in both texts, the crux of Herder's argument is precisely the question of Philoctetes' expression of pain. In the *Treatise* Herder concentrates on Philoctetes' piercing cry, and in *First Grove,* on his inspiring silence. The cry and its silencing are clearly crucial for Herder in staking his linguistic as well as aesthetic claims. This is precisely the strength of Herder's claim: howling the cry of pain and silencing it are essentially co-extensive. Both are expressions of pain.

Understanding this peculiar variation in the description of Philoctetes as a mere (and uncharacteristic) flaw in the rigor of Herder's philosophical argumentation would be an omission, nor should it be seen as intended to point at some unsolvable contradiction within Philoctetes himself. I take Herder's ambivalence here to reflect the very heart of his argument. The silent Philoctetes is not the negation of the crying one but his dialectical double. This point emerges when Herder criticizes Lessing's emphasis on the cry as the "keynote" of Sophocles' play, suggesting an antithetical argument: Philoctetes suffers wordlessly, only with a "suppressed "ah me!" "His lame foot, his grimacing face, his breast heaving as he sighs, his sides sunken with groans, his soft 'ah me!' Beyond this the poet does not go, and to forestall any exaggeration of expression, he has Philoctetes drift into unconsciousness with the pain! He has suffered so much, summoned his strength for so long, that he is beside himself" (*First Grove* 56). But Herder's repudiation of the cry does not amount to a rejection of Philoctetes' expression as such. On the contrary, what is so striking about Herder's claim here is that silence and heroic suppression disclose no less than does the terrible cry. Philoctetes' attempts to stifle his cry of pain, appear in Herder's interpretation as another form of expressing pain. Herder's emphasis in *First Grove,* is precisely on Philoctetes' subdued silence. The convulsed body and silently clenched lips are perhaps a negation of the cry but never a repudiation of expression: "The restraint, the agonized self-mastery, the long, silent struggles with his torment, which are finally ended with a stolen ὤ μοι! μοι!—these are drawn out, they creep, and they are the keynote of the entire scene . . . and it is a long, whole, complete act that fills my soul—not by uttering the cry but by suppressing it" (*First Grove* 58).

Sympathy

Despite the obvious differences between the two figures of Philoctetes—crying and silent—they are significantly linked: both imply the problem of sympathy. Sympathy is also a predominant issue in Sophocles' account of the myth. The problem at the heart of Sophocles' play is that of sympathy or the lack of it. To begin with, the problem of sympathy is not only pertinent to Philoctetes insofar as his abandonment is concerned. The experience of indifference to pain resonates with the circumstances in which he received his magic bow and arrows, the reason for Odysseus' voyage to the island. When Heracles is poisoned by Deianeira's dress, his skin torn and his bones exposed, he seeks help to end his tortured life. However, no one is willing to help. No one besides Philoctetes. He builds a funeral pyre, lights the fire, and frees Heracles from his pain.[40] In return, Heracles gives him his magic bow and arrows. This story presents Philoctetes as a man who has gained his invincible weapon by showing compassion. And it is he of all people who is left to suffer on his own.[41] Against this background, Odysseus represents an absence of sympathy, whereas Neoptolemus changes in the course of the play, eventually turning his back to Odysseus and his plot and becoming compassionate and faithful to Philoctetes and his pain. Neoptolemus' transformation takes place around the middle of the play, when he witnesses one of Philoctetes' terrible pain attacks: this is when Neoptolemus begins to develop deep feelings toward him: "A strange compassion for him comes upon me,/which I first felt, not now, but long before" (*Sophocles, Philoc.* 965), as well as a piercing guilt: "the turmoil I am in. . . . /I made a shameful error" (899, 1248). Neoptolemus' moral transformation proceeds as his feeling of sympathy deepens, revealing his true nature: "Everything is offensive," he tells Philoctetes, "when a man/departs from his own nature and does wrong" (903–904). He then confesses his and Odysseus' fraudulent scheme and finally convinces Odysseus to rescue Philoctetes—and the latter to agree to be rescued—from the island (with the faithful help of Heracles). The story ends with Philoctetes being cured and helping the Greeks win the war.[42]

Herder summons the figure of Philoctetes in his two above mentioned texts not only as representative of a man in terrible pain but also as a figure whose extreme suffering forcefully raises the problem of sympathy. In the *Treatise*, Philoctetes' cries yield a unique structure of echoes of sympathy throughout the whole of nature. In *First Grove*, his agony is analyzed in the theatrical context where the problem of sympathy arises between Philoctetes' suffering and the audience's feelings for him. Although perhaps not immediately obvious, Herder's two accounts and accordingly, the two figures of Philoctetes, crying and silent, remain in fact very close to one another: both present him as an exemplary figure whose pain is so extreme that it becomes unbearable, and both accounts scrutinize the expression of this pain in the context of the question of others' sympathy toward it. This remains Herder's focal point when Philoctetes screams in his solitude in the *Treatise*, but also when he stands strong, silently suppressing his terrible pain in *First Grove*. The question of sympathy arises as inherently bound up with pain's different forms of expression, so that both silent endurance and howling it out like an animal turn out to be two sides of the very same coin. In neither of these texts, however, does Herder discuss sympathy as a feeling or emotion toward another's pain and suffering. Sympathy for Herder is not something we feel *about* someone else or *toward* him. He describes sympathy, rather, as thoroughly physical: we literally feel-with another's pain by way of experiencing it in our very body.

In his description of the expressive structure of the original, natural language of sensation in the *Treatise*, Herder associates between the immediacy of the expression of pain and a corresponding immediacy of the natural sympathy it calls forth. The primal language of sensation offers a model of sympathy and compassion that prevails in the natural world and is constituted by the relationship between pain and its expression. It is this natural structure or, perhaps, the structure of pain itself, that releases the individual's painful sensations from their state of containment. Here Herder compares the primal cry of pain to the striking of the string of a musical instrument whose sound naturally provokes sympathetic reverberations:

> This is how little nature has created us as isolated rocks [abgesonderte Steinfelsen], as egoistic monads! Even the finest instrument strings [Saiten] of animal feeling (I have to use this metaphor because I know no better for the mechanism of feeling bodies!)—even these strings, whose sound and straining [Klang und Anstrengung] does not come from volition and slow deliberation at all. . . . [T]hese are directed in their whole play, even without the consciousness of foreign sympathy, at an expression [Äußerung] to other creatures. The struck string performs its natural duty [Naturpflicht]: it sounds!, it calls to a similarly feeling Echo—even when none is there, even when it does not hope or expect to be answered by one. (*Treatise* 65–66/*AS* 697–698)

Herder here describes the original state in which man and animal maintain a natural, joint linguistic accord, in terms of a system of musical strings. In Herder's metaphor, the striking of the strings is not the result of a voluntary linguistic act, expressing a propositional utterance that turns pain into linguistic "content." For Herder, this original sympathy is inaugurated by a much more basic and far-reaching transmission of the very sensation of pain itself: an immediate, physical externalization of pain from the body by means of sound, that is, the cry or the breath. The striking of the string is entirely mechanical, as are the reverberations of other strings that are touched by the sound waves of the original cry and resonate it in turn. This is why Herder argues that the cry does not depend on the existence of an addressee. Instead, we have a material, mechanical transmission whose inner motivating force consists of the very act of transmission itself, nothing more (this is what Herder means when he explains the cry of pain as a mere "externalization" of the pain's sensation). The sounds of pain, now scattered in the shared natural kingdom, are at the same time a distribution of pain itself, a sensation no longer belonging to an individual, suffering creature but one that is shared by all and becomes a communal sensation. In other words, with the cry, pain is transformed from a singular, subjective sensation to a potentially communal one, and it then necessarily follows that pain induces a similar communal feeling of sympathy. Although Herder's description of sympathy appears only a few lines after his reference to Philoctetes, it is clear that he puts forth a stark mirror image: natural, immediate, communal sympathy on the one hand, and the aloof turning away of Philoctetes' companions who leave him alone on the island, where there is only nature to echo his solitary cries.[43]

With this, Herder aligns with the eighteenth-century understanding of sympathy, especially as argued by Adam Smith, David Hume, and Jean-Jacques Rousseau.[44] One interesting case to consider in this respect is Hume's theory of sympathy. In his *Treatise of Human Nature* (1738–1740), Hume describes what he calls the moral "force of sympathy" in very similar terms to those of Herder. Hume argues for an inherent similarity in the structures of all human minds, feelings, and operations—a similarity so strong that no human mind can be "actuated by any affection, of which all others are not, in some degree, susceptible." Just like Herder, Hume uses a musical metaphor: "As in strings equally wound up, the motion of one communicates itself to the rest; so all the affections readily pass from one person to another, and beget correspondent movements in every human creature."[45] Herder's description of this sympathy is remarkable:

> As alone and individual and exposed to every hostile storm of the universe as it seems, it is not alone; it stands allied with the whole of nature! [es steht mit der ganzen Natur im Bunde!], delicately strung, but nature has hidden [verborgen] in these strings sounds which, stimulated and

> encouraged, awaken other equally delicately built creatures in turn, and can communicate sparks [Funken] to a remote heart, as though through an invisible chain, so that it feels for this unseen creature. (*Treatise* 66/ *AS* 698)[46]

The strength of this passage rests in its locus being in nature rather than in human society. Here, as opposed to later parts of the text, Herder relates to humans as being still integral to the natural world. Moreover, he suggests that the animal mechanism of feeling is necessary for sympathy. The striking of the string generates a natural sympathetic reverberation that brings all creatures together, a feeling of sympathy that crosses the boundaries between species, between human and animal.[47] The link Herder makes between communication and the word *Funken*, or spark, is significant: the sympathetic, natural communication emerges from a mechanical transmission in which a physical spark elicits other sparks in a "remote heart." The reverberation demonstrated in the string metaphor suggests a complex form of echoing: not merely a weaker variant of the original cry, the resonating sound gives rise to a much more active composite of tones, so that one strike or one cry of pain has the power to yield an expansive configuration of corresponding reverberations.

In *Outlines of a Philosophy of the History of Man*, Herder offers yet another version of this structure of sympathy, this time focusing on humans' unique sympathetic ability to participate in the suffering of other creatures.[48] The human being's heightened sensitivity (which Herder describes with reference to human nerves) allows "every part of his vibrating frame" to take part in and share the feelings of others, "in the degree necessary to the creature" (*Ideas*, Book 4 99). What stands out here is Herder's shift of attention from a natural to a human frame of reference: the human being—and in this he is unlike other living creatures—can adjust the *degree* of his sympathy to that "necessary" to the suffering creature. This formulation can be understood in a variety of ways, of which I here touch on only one: while a human feeling of sympathy is natural, even mechanical (the product of his nervous structure), it can also accommodate itself to the specific suffering it encounters. Although Herder does not state it explicitly, this passage seems to suggest that human sympathy turns not only toward its own species but is capable of hearing and responding to the natural world as a whole.

The "finest instrument strings of animal feeling," in Herder's words, originate not in volition, deliberation, or any type of consciousness but are nevertheless directed toward the induction of strong natural sympathy (*Treatise* 65–66/ *AS* 697–698). This pain-based sympathy does not result from designative, propositional, and communicative language; it stems, rather, from the bare sounding and resounding of pain itself. These sounds, together with the intimate connections they arouse among their bearers, form the groundworks for a community founded on sympathy. The "tiring breath, the semi-groan, which dies so movingly on the lip distorted by pain," is at this stage in the text not yet separate "from all its living helpers" (*Treatise* 68/*AS* 700). Language, intertwined with the natural shared community, has not yet attained the distance required for the production of signs or ciphers, as Herder calls them (*Treatise* 68/*AS* 700). In Herder's narrative, language at this stage is not yet human; however, in terms of the compassion and sympathy it affords, it can be seen as a blueprint for humanness.[49]

Herder proposes that we consider this unique linguistic configuration of expression and its sympathetic reverberation as an immediate, "clear law of nature": "Here is a sensitive being which can enclose none of its lively sensations within itself, which in the first moment of surprise, even without volition and intention, has to express each of them in sound" [first formulation]. "Do not have sensation for yourself alone, but may your feeling resound!" [dein Gefühl töne!] [second formulation]. "May your sensation resound for your species in a single way, and therefore be perceived by all, as by a single one, with sympathy!" [mitfühlend vernommen!] [third formulation] (*Treatise* 66/*AS* 698). The first formulation of the law describes the suffering creature who is unable to contain the painful sensations within the confines of his body, when pain takes over and compels him to violently express it in cries and howls. The second formulation is a variant of the first, substituting the descriptive tone with an imperative: the suffering creature *must* express its sensations in sound. The imperative to express in the law's second formulation becomes a "blessing" in the third formulation where Herder associates the cry of pain with its sympathetic echo. Taking Herder's natural law to be the foundation of what can be read as a preliminary moral conjecture, an interesting structure emerges. The first two formulations of the law foreground the imperative to express pain, to convey it by way of an immediate sounding—and not, as expected from the formulation of moral law, the duty to respond to the cry of the other. The third formulation, in effect, is a "blessing" that emerges when the first two formulations are taken together. The imperative evolves into a blessing when the single creature's expression of pain encounters its echo and learns that "it is not alone." Put otherwise, the natural becomes moral when an immediate, instinctive, and individual expression of pain transforms into the very foundation of a community. The uniqueness of this transition from the natural to the moral lies in Herder's emphasis on the suffering creature's *consciousness* of his belonging, so that the cry of pain becomes a way (perhaps the only way) in which the creature discovers that he is allied, belongs, and sparks responses.

Herder puts forth an interesting formulation in which the natural and the moral are not at odds; rather, the grounds of one of the most difficult paradoxes of human nature are continuous with one another so that the natural becomes the moral and vice versa. Herder's laws of sympathy are natural laws, that is, they obey the necessary principles governing nature and in that sense, they are followed involuntarily (like, say, the law of gravity); however, since they involve sympathy and a feeling for the other, they are also formulated as moral laws ("May your sensation resound . . . [and] be perceived by all, as by a single one, with sympathy!)" [*Treatise* 66/*AS* 698]). *Nature* too, has a twofold meaning: on the one hand, it denotes the natural world as opposed to human society and in the *Treatise* includes human beings as well as animals (or humans when they were "already" animals, as Herder puts it). On the other hand, nature designates what Herder takes to be *human nature,* that is, the essential condition of our being human, that without which we are not human. In this sense, our belonging to nature (in the *Treatise*) is imperative in our own nature as human beings (in *First Grove*). In both cases, this nature has to do with our animal being and what it endows us with, namely, our immediate reaction of sympathy for suffering others. So that when a wailing, suffering animal or a "man with a death rattle" express their anguish, there is "nothing before me but the spectacle of a man wracked by convulsions, in sympathy with whom I too very nearly feel palpitations, of a whimpering man whose 'ah!' cuts through my heart" (*First Grove* 78). Herder accentuates the heart yet again when he writes in the *Treatise,* immediately after his description of the moral/natural laws, that the cry of pain stirs up feelings in other creatures and "communicate[s] sparks to a remote heart [einem entfernten Herzen Funken mitteilen können], as though through an invisible chain, so that it feels for this unseen creature" (*Treatise* 66/*AS* 698).[50] This is why Herder insists on describing these laws of nature as "immediate," that is un-mediated or direct (*unmittelbares Naturgesetz*). Herder's use of the term "species" (*Geschlecht*) in this context is noteworthy. He is well aware (and this is further developed later on in the *Treatise*) that the cries of a suffering animal are received, and responded to, by its own species. Here, however, when he is still describing the primary language of sensation, the species-specific cry is received and felt by all ("deine Empfindung töne deinem Geschlecht einartig und werde also von allen wie von *einem* mitfühlend vernommen!" [*AS* 698]). Confronted with cries of pain and suffering, the human heart is touched with compassion and sympathy for the suffering human or animal. Those who remain untouched Herder describes, as "feelingless barbarians":

> Since our natural sounds are destined for the expression of passion [Leidenschaft], it is natural *that they also become the elements of all moving* [Rührung] *[of another person]!* Who is there who, faced with a shaking, whining tortured person, with a moaning dying person, and even with a groaning farm animal when its whole machine is suffering,

> is not touched to his heart by this “Ah!”? [dies Ach nicht zu Herzen dringe?]. Who is such a feelingless barbarian? The more harmoniously the sensitive string-play is woven even in the case of animals with other animals, the more even these feel with one another; their nerves come to a similar tension [Spannung], their souls to a similar pitch [gleichmäßigen Ton], they really share each other’s pain mechanically [leiden würklich mechanisch mit]. (*Treatise* 72/*AS* 705–706)

In this description, nature responds to pain mechanically, but this has no implications for the moral value of the response. The trembling string and its echo physically tie together the whole of nature through the substratum of intense pain. When human language is still in its birth pangs, when it has not yet developed, we feel for or sympathize with the other’s suffering all the more strongly and directly.[51] Addressing Diderot’s description of the blind person, Herder writes, “Horror and pain shoots through his limbs, his inner nerve structure feels the breaking and destruction in sympathy [sein innrer Nervenbau fühlt Bruch und Zerstörung mit]; the death rattle [Todeston] sounds.[52] That is the *bond of this natural language*!” [Das ist das Band dieser Natursprache!] (*Treatise* 73/*AS* 706). Herder’s reference to the blind here is suggestive insofar as beyond emphasizing the moral dictum inherent to the cry, it also accentuates its sonic dimension (in contrast to the visual presence of a pained creature). The blind person does not merely hear the cry but he also feels it in every limb of his body. The inner breaking is thus *mit*-felt, that is, felt-with.[53]

The bond of sympathy is fractured, however, when distinctly human language arises. Sympathy is traded for communication, a form of communication very different from that conducted in natural language. In the pure linguistic sense (which governs the remainder of the treatise), human language is a stronger and more advanced form of communication, based on concepts, abstractions, and the ability to think systematically; however, in all other respects, it appears to be weaker. The prefix “com-” of communication marks something quite different from the “com-” of comm-unity, and com-passion. Herder’s presentation thus abides by a fundamental premise of the Enlightenment—namely, that the advantages of rationality and logos exact a price. In Herder’s philosophical system, this price is, among other things, the inability to sympathize, especially in the political context. “Letters for the Advancement of Humanity” (1793–97) elaborates on this political price: “Certainly a dangerous gift, power without kindness, incentive slyness without understanding. . . . In novels we cry for a butterfly whose wings get wetted by the rain; in conversations we bubble over with great sentimental dispositions—and for this moral corruption of our species, from which all evil arises, we have no eye.”[54] When humans elevate themselves above nature on account of their achievement of language, they gain their freedom, but at the same time they forfeit the natural, intuitive part of their ability for sympathy, solicitude, and compassion. The degeneration of the capacity for compassion marks the point at which Herder parts from the primordial language of sensation for the sake of its decisive development into a distinctly human language.

The story of Philoctetes and his disturbing abandonment immediately comes to mind. Philoctetes' cry in the *Treatise* generates an exceedingly different response from the one he received from his fellow soldiers in Sophocles' rendering of the story. Instead of expressing an immediate, natural sympathy or solidarity, Philoctetes' companions are disgusted and appalled by the wound and especially by Philoctetes' ghastly expressions of pain. Instead of eliciting a communal reverberation of feeling, Philoctetes finds himself alone on a desert island, in the sole company of his own grief and cries (*Sophocles, Philoc.* 282–283).

Neoptolemus' moral reform in the third act of the play provides us with a different model of sympathy:[55] Philoctetes' cries do not drive the young boy away; rather, it is precisely their inarticulate, immediate nature that transforms Neoptolemus' feeling for Philoctetes and brings out what he later calls the "natural" bud of sympathy in him. In sympathy he discovers, in other words, his own "true nature" (*Sophocles, Philoc.* 904). The figure of Neoptolemus aligns here with Herder's account of sympathy in the *Treatise*, offering an alternative to customary accounts of the solipsism of the pained, suffering individual whose isolation is grounded in, and manifested by, the essential inability to "share" one's pain with others in language (i.e., the "unshareable" nature of pain according to Scarry). In Herder's alternative structure, represented by Neoptolemus, it is precisely the immediacy of Philoctetes' cry, rather than a mediated, accurate concept or statement, that enables true feeling and sympathy. Here Philoctetes' "Ah! Ah!" and Neoptolemus' feeling of sympathy come together in the *Treatise*, where Herder wonders, "Who is there who, faced with a shaking, whining tortured person . . . is not touched to his heart by this 'Ah!' "? (*Treatise* 72/*AS* 705). In what might seem to be Herder's ideal or naive portrayal of primordial morality, Philoctetes' Ah! is immediately answered with feeling, by a law of nature. In this conception, when an animal or human being howls in pain, we do not, and cannot, recoil from their suffering, reflect in doubt, or fail in any other way to fully grasp the pain (think of them as "other minds," that is), or even worse, grasp it but be unable to bear it.[56] Rather, we feel the pain with them, in each tiniest nerve of our very being (body and soul), because the sufferer's struck strings have immediately affected and moved ours.[57]

Herder's discussion of Philoctetes in *First Grove* seems to suggest a similar emphasis on sympathy but with an important difference: if in the *Treatise* sympathy emerges from the immediate animal cry of pain, in *First Grove* it issues not from Philoctetes' cry, but rather from his sturdy, subdued silence. Recounting the story in chapter 5 of *First Grove*, Herder focuses on the way in which Philoctetes' words, as well as silences, bodily gestures, and dumbstruck gazes, forcefully affect the audience of Sophocles' play. He describes in detail how sympathy is first "planted" in the spectators' hearts by the chorus and later developed into a deep overarching feeling for the hero's suffering. Herder argues that the audience's sympathy for Philoctetes does not stem from the hero's crying, howling, or any other excessive expressions of pain, but arises, rather, from the opposite: "How I feel for Philoctetes! But for Philoctetes the screamer? I feel nothing yet! I feel for Philoctetes the hero, the Greek, the nobleman" (*First Grove* 75). In order for sympathy to be generated and fostered, no clamorous cries are needed. On the contrary, the deep compassionate feeling for Philoctetes' suffering is triggered by his subdued "Ah!," by his admirable effort to suffocate the anguished cry for which his bodily instincts yearn.

In the subsequent description of the unique nature of sympathy generated by the dramatic medium, *First Grove* converges with the *Treatise* by way of a common metaphor:

> With physical pain I cannot but sympathize physically: that is, sympathy causes a similarly painful tension to be produced in my fibers; I suffer the pain in my own body. . . .[T]he cry of distress, the convulsion passes through my every limb with a shudder; I feel it myself; the same spasmodic movements manifest themselves in me, as if I were a string tuned to the same pitch. (*First Grove* 77)

Here we find the same wording Herder uses a few years later in the *Treatise* where the animal feeling is described as "the finest instrument strings [feinsten Saiten]" and the pained 'Ah!' brings the animal's nerves "to a similar tension [Spannung], their souls to a similar pitch" [gleichmäßige Ton] (*Treatise* 65, 72/*AS* 697, 705). What is so remarkable in both these texts is Herder's emphasis on the physical, bodily sphere in which sympathy emerges. Philoctetes' silent yet tormented body does not inspire an emotion or feeling toward his suffering, nor does it provide a reason for us, the audience, to be sympathetic. Similar to the animal in the *Treatise*, the theater spectator responds to the cry of pain much like to the suppressed "Ah!" with his entire physique, feeling Philoctetes' pain as if it were part of his own body.

It is not a shudder-*for* someone else, or a feeling in reference *to* his suffering; this suffering becomes my very own shuddering, my own pain: "Woe is me! My nerves twitch!" (*First Grove* 77). Herder's musical trope bears this out: my feeling-with the other's pain is as vehement "as if I were a string tuned to the same pitch." The moment of intense pain reveals something crucial: rather than being distanced by pain, onlooker and sufferer are brought together by it. They discover (by way of experience, not knowledge) that their strings are tuned to the same pitch, that they are, so to speak, sympathetic to one another in their very being. The experience of pain has, therefore, the unique power to reveal something about our coexistence rather than about our dissociation or the unbridgeable gap between us. In light of the well-established view regarding pain's isolating and destructive nature and the essential doubt it plants in us, creating a sense of irreconcilable distance—Herder's alternative stands out clear and distinct.

In Herder's approach to sympathy, an important difference between the crying and the silent Philoctetes emerges. Sympathy in the *Treatise* is purely mechanical; although its strength lies in that it testifies to the similarity, even kinship, between all creatures, it is in no way voluntary or intentional. The "sensitive machine" responds mechanically; its strings and fibers move automatically. The silent, noble Philoctetes of *First Grove*, on the other hand, presents an entirely different conception of sympathy. Here sympathy is constituted not by the cry of pain or any similarity between sufferer and audience; it is produced by the effective dynamics between the intensity of pain and Philoctetes' ability to contain it. Consequently, restraining the pain and curbing the cry become the source of a growing, vigorous feeling of sympathy. Moreover, the mechanical response apparatus in the *Treatise* is replaced here with a crucial interruption or suspension in which pain is restrained and the hero is silent. This moment opens a breach (crucially missing in the mechanical account) from which a decision can be made: sympathy is now not compulsory but volitional, it is conditioned by the silence that allows the space necessary to reflect, to take a moral stand and decide to feel for the suffering hero instead of merely being passively moved by his cry. This choice constitutes the point at which sympathetic (animal) instinct turns into (human) moral feeling.

The Principle of Expression

Although so far I have been primarily concerned with the natural language of sensation that opens Herder's text, the structure of the *Treatise* seems to reveals an apparently different picture. After only nine pages Herder moves to discussing the predominant linguistic structure in the *Treatise*, namely, human, reflective language, to which chapter 3 is devoted. But first, it is important to consider the relationship between the two languages—between sensation and reflection—a problem that can benefit from Isaiah Berlin's famous distinction between the Enlightenment and what he calls the "Counter-Enlightenment." In his *Vico and Herder* (1980), Berlin establishes Herder as a critic of the Enlightenment by attributing three main principles to his thought: populism (the principle of belonging), pluralism (the belief in the incommensurability of values and ideals in different cultures and societies), and expressionism. The last term refers very broadly to expression in general while at the same time emphasizing the importance of self-expression, which accentuates the crucial role of expression in the self-realization of the entangled, at times conflicting, essence of human beings. This self-realization, Berlin argues, still with reference to Herder, is the "richest and most harmonious form of self-expression that all creatures, whether or not they are aware of it, live for."[58]

Charles Taylor relies on Berlin's argument and develops it in various texts, in which he renames Berlin's expressionism as "expressivism," a term suggested to him by Berlin himself in a private conversation, to avoid confusion with the early twentieth-century movement.[59] Taylor interprets Herder's theory of language against the background of the latter's criticism of designative linguistic structures such as those of Condillac and Locke. Even in its most factual, mundane functions, Taylor claims, our language is never limited to its mere designative dimension in referring to existing states of affairs: "We experience our essentially human emotions not primarily in describing, but in expressing them. Language also serves to express/realize ways of feeling without identifying them in description. We often give expression of our feelings in talking about something else."[60] According to Taylor, Herder's principle of expression demonstrates a rejection of the dichotomy between meaning and being, and more important, incorporates an idea of a "self-defining subjectivity," in which the realization of human essence is achieved by way of self-realization, a realization of "something which unfolds from himself, is his own realization, and is first made determinate in that realization."[61] Similarly, Forster emphasizes the challenges Herder poses to the dualistic Enlightenment model in which meanings feature as "separable and autonomous from whatever material, perceptible expressions they may happen to receive in language, and of language as merely a means to their communication which is quite inessential to their actual existence."[62] This principle of expression (demonstrated most explicitly in Herder's theory of language but also in his ideas about history, nationalism, and poetry) has become the crux (at least, the most famous one) of Berlin's argument that Herder is first and foremost a critic of the Enlightenment's core values.

Berlin's and Taylor's stimulating discussions importantly drew attention to and awakened interest in Herder's thought. Including Herder under the rubric of Counter-Enlightenment, however, also problematically reinforces a dichotomizing use of the categories of Enlightenment and Counter-Enlightenment in considering Herder's ideas. Berlin's and Taylor's interpretations led them to ignore some of Herder's own, at times very explicit statements expressing his commitment to some fundamental principles of the Enlightenment.[63] However, a close reading of Herder reveals that a characterization of his Counter-Enlightenment position should refer not only to his treatment of the human language of reflection and awareness, but also (perhaps even more so) to his analysis of the primary language of sensation.

It is interesting to observe that in their attempt to "rescue" Herder from the grip of the Enlightenment, both interpreters choose not to dwell on the beginning of the *Treatise* and its detailed account of the original language of sensation, establishing their argument regarding expression and the Counter-Enlightenment almost exclusively on human, reflective language. In doing so, Berlin and Taylor fall into their own pit: on the one hand, they disregard Herder's explicit commitment to the ideas of the Enlightenment; on the other, they base their principle of expression solely on Herder's account of human language, which he explicitly describes as opposing the natural language of sensations.

I suggest, therefore, that we take Berlin's and Taylor's emphasis on expression as the essential and determining principle governing Herder's view of distinctly *human* language and rethink its importance, taking into account the primordial language of sensation as well. Here I might appear to stretch Berlin's and Taylor's claims a bit beyond where they wanted them to go but I remain faithful to the heart of their argument, namely that, as Taylor puts it, "language can't be confined to the activity of talking about things"; rather, it expresses and realizes a wide array of feeling and emotion that words cannot convey.[64] This argument refers, of course, to Herder's conception of human language, but its main features are clearly and crucially present in his notion of the primary language of sensation as well. This argument becomes even more interesting and suggestive when we notice that most of Herder's interpreters tend to discuss the *Treatise* starting from its second part, almost completely neglecting the beginning of the text with its focus on the language of sensation. Once we include this part as integral to Herder's treatise text, we realize that the term "expressionism" (or expressivism) not only articulates the contribution and originality of Herder's *Treatise* against the background of the Enlightenment but is also present in an explicit and powerful form in the very first pages of the *Treatise*.

While Herder is clearly not an epitome of the Enlightenment it would be inaccurate to read his work as a wholesale repudiation of the Enlightenment's core values. It was Ernst Cassirer who put this plainly when writing that although Herder seemed to be a resolute opponent of the ideas of the Enlightenment, he was frank enough to admit how important it was to him "as long as it was wise enough not to claim to be everything."[65] If we want to read "with" Herder rather than taking an extraneous perspective, we must carefully follow his intricate dialectics in which the "counter" elements emerge from *within* the ideas of the Enlightenment and not as their opposites. Herder's position is indeed unique and radical, as Berlin and Taylor rightfully established, but this uniqueness inheres in Herder's ability to challenge the ideas of the Enlightenment from within, to undermine them while still remaining faithful to its central tenets. The task at hand is now to approach Herder's theory of language from neither an Enlightenment nor a Counter-Enlightenment position, but to release the hold of these categories and attempt to follow Herder's own footsteps in singling out what distinguishes his approach to language and its origin from a third perspective, namely, the human.

Philoctetes' cry reveals not merely his animal-being but also the essential animality that forms the basis of his very humanity. In Herder's argument, this animality concerns not only the suffering creature but also, and perhaps foremost, the agonized onlooker. "Whether the whimpering man gripped by a seizure is Philoctetes does not concern me," Herder writes; "he is an animal, just as I am; he is a human being: human pain agitates my nervous system, just as it does when I see a dying animal, a man with the death rattle, a creature in torment who feels as I do. . . . Nature, my animal being suffers within me, for I see and hear an animal of my species suffer" (*First Grove* 77). Philoctetes' distinct characteristics (his wound, pain, abandonment, and so forth) appear on stage only in order to be stripped away and to expose the underlying essential being. Articulating the internal voice of the observer, Herder asserts how Philoctetes the mythical figure makes way for Philoctetes the animal, which in turn echoes and reveals the observer's own animality; but this is, importantly, a *moral* animality, since the cry of pain reveals that "he is an animal, just as I am"; our strings vibrate at a similar pitch and his tortured body literally moves mine.

This illuminates the importance of the link between *First Grove* and the *Treatise* which are now revealed to be resonating one another rather than being mere opposites. In both texts, Herder introduces an evocative perspective on pain and its outcry, both manifesting a singular power to uncover a shared, communal essence between sufferer and onlooker. This point is borne out by another paragraph from *First Grove*, especially when we read it against the background of the *Treatise*. Referring to Lessing's claim that our emotions do not follow or obey any general rules, Herder remarks: "Here the law lies in my immediate feeling itself, namely in that feeling which is farthest removed from general principles, that feeling with which I am endowed as an animal capable of sympathy" (*First Grove* 78). Though sympathy operates according to laws, these are inner laws ordained and obeyed by the immediacy of feeling. Herder's law of immediate feeling in *First Grove* aligns with the laws of nature he described in the *Treatise*. This is manifest in the dual significance of Herder's use of the term "nature": if "nature" in the *Treatise* seemed to refer to the natural world in the narrow sense, which subsequently becomes detached from the distinctly human realm, *First Grove* suggests that "nature" also signifies "essence," and the essence of the human being is, in fact, his animal being.

3

Language and Attention

Herder on Besonnenheit

Herder's Two Languages: Sensation and Reflection

In my interpretation of Herder's *Treatise,* the language of sensations and "artificial" human language are contradictory, much like Herder's two figures of Philoctetes—that is, not at all, or at least only on the face of it. Just as the crying Philoctetes and the silent Philoctetes are not mere opposites but bespeak a composite, so too, the two languages are not plainly distinct or separate, and definitely not mutually exclusive. Just as understanding Philoctetes means bearing in mind the two versions, his cry as well as his silence, so too in order to understand Herder's philosophy of language it is never enough to merely study the second part of the *Treatise,* which explicitly discusses human language. There is no silencing of the cry if there is no cry; there is no abstract, reflective human expression, if it were not for the immediate animal howl of pain accompanied by immediate sympathy. Language is "already" (*schon*) there from the start.

Before delving into the second part of the *Treatise* in which Herder treats human language, I would like to discuss briefly the relationship between the two languages. When Herder describes the development of human language, his argument takes a clearly anthropological tone: "artificial language," as he calls it, or language founded on arbitrary signs "dries out the river of feeling" to replace the original language of expressive immediacy. Herder attributes this artificiality to what he calls the "civilized (*bürgerliche*) manner of life," which, having replaced the language of nature, brings about a critical change that has "dammed, dried out, and drained off the flood and sea of passions" (*Treatise* 66/*AS* 698–699). What Herder sees as the overcoming of emotion, specifically pain, with the emergence of human language, is thus structured as *suppression* more than *alleviation.* This suppression, however, is not complete. Herder repeatedly uses violent expressions to describe the diverse ways in which the primordial, affective language of sensations continues to appear and reappear in different guises to remind us of the hidden origin of reflective human language.[1] He specifically chooses expressions referring to the capacity of human language to neutralize the "sea of passions," the impetuous storms of feeling and the sudden inundation of emotions—all of which reassume their rights from the depths of original human language and continue to resound within their "mother tongue" through emphases (*Akzente*) and intonations: "The sudden accession of joy or happiness, pain and misery when they dig deep furrows into the soul, an overpowering feeling of revenge, despair, fury, fright, horror, etc.—all announce themselves, and each one differently according to its kind" (*Treatise* 67/*AS* 699). Herder claims, thus, that the original language poses a continual challenge to human language but cannot wholly overpower it.

Another consequence of the formative engagement between the natural language of sensations and human language is that, to quote Herder in *Fragments*, the more exact language becomes, the more reduced is its emotional richness (*Fragments* 33). Herder's principal concern here is not merely the decline of the expressive quality of language but the radical dilution of the fundamental human capacity to sympathize with the pain of others: when deprived of the immediacy of expression, human language also loses its moral infrastructure (so central to the first pages of the *Treatise*). In making this claim, however, Herder in fact suggests a much broader contention: language not merely represents an inner world of emotions and feelings that mysteriously exists prior to its linguistic expression, but rather it constitutes the very essence of that internal universe. There can, consequently, be no categorical separation between the linguistic capacities and the emotional and moral aptitude.

Herder's account of human language in the second part of the *Treatise* is in this sense an argument pertaining to the nature of human beings as such. The two issues, language and humanity, are not only inherently linked; for Herder, they are one and the same thing. This is why in describing the transition from the original language of sensations into human, reflective language, Herder does not focus merely on a differentiation between the two languages, or on the ways in which the animal, sensual language of immediacy is inadequate for humans insofar as the latter are social animals (such an approach would be similar to Rousseau or Condillac). Herder approaches the problem of language from an entirely different perspective, offering an account of the essence of the human being. Whereas the first part of the text begins with the words "Schon als Tier" (already as an animal), the second part is dominated by different versions of the phrase "als der Mensch ein Mensch war" (when the human being was a human being): "The invention of language is hence as natural for him as is his being a human being!" [Erfindung der Sprache ist ihm also so natürlich, als er ein

Mensch ist!] (*Treatise* 87/*AS* 722).[2] However, notwithstanding Herder's emphatic denunciation of positions arguing for the language of sensations as the origin of human language, and in spite of the more pro-Enlightenment position which we might expect, Herder's argument boldly implies that human language is not established by reason or the power of abstract thought; it does not come to satisfy a communicative or social need, or function as a means to represent and transmit any form of propositional content. Human language is also not some external characteristic or element added on to the original human animal; it is not about the physics of the human mouth or the ability to produce articulate sounds; it is not a mere animal cry of sensations and also does not amount to an imitation of natural sounds. Least of all, Herder argues, is language a communal understanding (*Einverständnis*) or arbitrary convention (*Treatise* 90/*AS* 725).

Instead, according to Herder, language is the way in which the human being orients himself in the world, positioning himself by way of an act of simultaneous differentiation and relation. Language marks how humankind comes to be in tune with the world, finds itself in it. Man's first word is, therefore, neither communicative nor referential but expresses a relationship with the world (and not necessarily with other human beings), so that with language, the world comes to belong to the human being, to matter to it.[3] The human being finds himself, however, not only in relation to the world or his surroundings, but also and more importantly in relation to himself. The appearance of both world and self is figured linguistically.

Besonnenheit: Awareness and Reflection

Herder names the singularly human characteristic that immediately also becomes the essence of language *Besonnenheit*. This term, a combination of intentionality, awareness, and reflection, is difficult to render in English. For Herder, Besonnenheit marks the distinctive disposition of the human being in relation to the animal, permitting the former to transcend primitive, instinctive, animal existence. Humans, contrary to animals, are creatures of awareness in virtue of the "freely effective positive force" of their soul, with Besonnenheit as an orientation and accommodation of all forces in a central direction (*Treatise* 85/*AS* 719). Nowhere does Herder provide an explanation for how this special capacity comes about, yet he treats it as *the* factor defining the human being's nature and entity.[4] Herder can be criticized here in the same terms in which he himself criticized Condillac: he assumes what he sets out to prove. Herder introduces Besonnenheit following a lengthy discussion of the distinction between what he calls "the life sphere" (*Kreis* or life circle) of humans and of animals. This type of explanation bears out Herder's keenness to distance himself from an account in which language is a mere addition to the animal that will then become a "speaking-animal." Instead, Besonnenheit encapsulates the delicate shift in the configuration of humans' relation to the world, compared to that of animals. This difference will become a manifestation of human linguistic capabilities.

The life of an animal is concentrated within the limited "life circle" into which it is born and in which it dies. The only linguistic capacity it needs is immediate expression (for instance, of pain or of pleasure). This function is directly shared with those members of its own species that inhabit the same sphere: "The spider weaves with the art of Minerva; but all its art is also woven out in this narrow spinning-space; that is its world! How marvelous is the insect, and how narrow the circle of this effect!" (*Treatise* 78/*AS* 712). The narrowness of the animal world is not presented as a limitation or weakness on part of the animal. Herder makes a point of the "marvelousness" of animals' instinctive skills:

> When infinitely fine senses are confined to a small circle, to uniformity, and the whole remaining world is nothing for them, how they must penetrate! When forces of representation are confined to a small circle and endowed with an analogous sensuality, what effect they must have! And finally, when senses and representations are directed at a single point, what else can become of this but instinct? Hence these explain the sensitivity, the abilities, and the drives of the animals according to their kinds and levels. (*Treatise* 79/*AS* 713)

The narrower and more limited the animal's circle (to the effect that "the whole remaining world is nothing to them"), the more it manifests its mastery of that circle. It controls everything about it; its senses are sharp and activities accurate. Herder describes this marvel by using terms such as "attention" and "focus." The force of the animal and its mastery of its environment renders it a creature to which language is virtually unnecessary. The smaller its life sphere, the less language it requires. Herder describes animal language as a "ruling instinct," and he observes: "How little it must speak in order to be heard!" [Wie wenig darf er sprechen, daß er vernommen werde!] (*Treatise* 79/*AS* 714). Animals have, hence, "little or no language" (*Treatise* 80/*AS* 714).[5]

This sets the scene for Herder's introduction of human beings. However, the human enters not as a powerful master of nature or ruler of the natural hierarchy (as is customary in eighteenth-century texts about language or society). The human being appears as a weak, limited creature, very unlike the animal with its extraordinarily focused, sharp mastery: "The human being has no such uniform and narrow sphere where only a single sort of work awaits him; a world of occupations and destinies surrounds him. His senses and organization are not sharpened for a single thing; he has senses for everything and hence naturally for each particular thing weaker and duller senses" [stumpfere Sinne] (*Treatise* 79/*AS* 713). This is why humans are the weakest creatures: while they do not entirely belong to any specific life sphere they dominate an infinite number of such spheres. Humans therefore lack the perspicacity and determination of the life-orienting instinct typical of a narrow and specialized life sphere. The consonance between human and nature maintained in the first pages of the *Treatise* falls apart at precisely this point: animals' instincts, specifically constituted in relation to their narrow life circles, have no parallel in human beings.

Herder treats animal language as inseparable from other animal skills and drives; all are innate and immediately natural to the animal: "The bee hums just as it sucks, the bird sings just as it makes a nest" (*Treatise* 80/*AS* 714). The human being, in contrast, possesses nothing like such a natural language, as it is deprived of any instinctive drive; it is dumb, "merely set among animals, therefore, it is the most orphaned child of nature. Naked and bare, weak and needy, timid and unarmed" (*Treatise* 80/*AS* 714).[6] Herder, however, is not satisfied with understanding human essence as a mere negation of the animal's impressive skill. The human being cannot only be a weak, dispersed creature. Herder defines the essence of the human being not as a form of compensation for its weakness, dispersion of forces, and lack of natural instincts; the human being, for Herder, is never simply a weak animal working against its shortcomings. The nature of the human being has to be found elsewhere (*Treatise* 80–81/*AS* 715).

Herder defines humans' linguistic capabilities as emanating not from their animal being but rather from whatever it is that sets them apart as humans. This differentiating feature, however, is not presented as an additional element external to humans' instinctive animal being but lies rather in the inherent dissimilarity between humans' and animals' relations with their surroundings. The crux of this difference will turn out to be language. Herder begins the second section of the *Treatise* with a statement seemingly aligned with the Enlightenment approach to the issue: "If the human being had animal *senses,* then he would have no *reason;* for precisely his senses' strong susceptibility to stimulation, precisely the representations mightily pressing on him through them, would inevitably choke all cold awareness" [Besonnenheit] (*Treatise* 84/*AS* 718–719). Herder claims here that the characterization of the human being as rational is mutually exclusive with his definition as a sensing animal, since the animal's extreme sensitivity does not only clash with reason, but it also violently subjugates the human being's rational abilities by "choking" all possible awareness. This however is not where Herder's argument ends. He continues as follows: "But conversely . . . it was also inevitably the case that: If animal sensuality and restriction to a single point *fell away,* then a different creature came into being, *whose positive force expressed itself in a larger space, in accordance with finer organization, more clearly*, and which, separated and free, not only cognizes, wills, and effects, but also knows that it cognizes, wills, and effects. This creature is the human being" (*Treatise* 84/*AS* 719). Here we have a slightly different formulation: the human being is not categorically different from the animal (as the beginning of the *Treatise* clearly shows); its nature is constituted, rather, as different from the animal's sensual, instinctive, narrow focus, embodying an alternative form of perception and being in the world, a form that Herder describes as linguistic.

This marks the crucial turn in Herder's argument. It is precisely from man's weakness and deprivation (relative to instinctual animals) that his greatest power stems: human beings are the only creatures compelled to create language:[7] "The invention of language is hence as natural for him as is his being a human being!" (*Treatise* 87/*AS* 722).[8] With these claims, Herder distances himself from the simple, expressive model of immediacy featuring in the first part of the *Treatise* and replaces it with a more sophisticated, reflective structure in which humans, by dint of their being human, bring to bear their linguistic abilities in creating and expressing their unique relationship with their world. Herder's Besonnenheit is his way to explain how the human being compensates for his lack of animal focus, specificity, and sharpness of instinct. Besonnenheit's special combination of awareness, attention, and reflection allows the human being to master the unimaginable vastness of his life sphere, his expansive, multifarious world.

Herder repeatedly stresses that "reason is no compartmentalized, separately effective force," and Besonnenheit is consequently not a separate force that is added to the animal, turning it into a human being. Rather, Besonnenheit is an organization, orientation, and unfolding of all his other forces, abilities, perceptions, and reason and the human being "*must have it in the first condition in which he is a human being*" (*Treatise* 85/*AS* 719). Further on in the *Treatise*, Herder returns to his discussion of human and animal, adding yet another feature to the comparison: while the bee was always the same bee and its singular crafts always and essentially remain the same, the human being, by contrast, never stops *becoming* a human being. Besonnenheit turns the human soul into a "*force of steadily collecting*," continuously building and evolving. Thus the animal has always been and will always be a consummate, accomplished creature, whereas man is "never the *whole human being*; always in development, in progression, in process of perfection" (*Treatise* 130/*AS* 773).

Despite his inclination to define the human being by turning away from his description of animal being, Herder does not fully dismiss the presence of original language's expressive elements in human language. He points out, instead, how, in the framework of human language, they evolve through Besonnenheit. What Herder presents here is in fact an organic model in which the reflexive dimensions of language spring forth from their expressive origins. If we go back to the "classic" picture of the acute division between emotion and reason,

Besonnenheit offers an alternative to this binary. Human language contains emotive facets and needs not renounce them in order to evolve.[9] More important, applying this organic model, Herder in fact claims there is no inherent gap between the two languages, even though the "origin" of language (of a clearly affective nature) is manifestly divergent from the stage when it becomes distinctly human. Instead, Herder constructs a continuity between the two linguistic forms through his use of Besonnenheit, which is revealed as a force orienting the affective dimensions of language rather than substituting for them. Put differently, the origin of human language is not transcended but remains strongly present: original human-animal language is not replaced by a more advanced instrument of expression but is reorganized and reoriented so as to establish as well as manifest its human character.

Before I continue with a more elaborate interpretation of the Herder's Besonnenheit, I would like to dedicate a few words to the similarity between Herder's theory and Wittgenstein's later philosophy of language. Herder's argument, that human language is not to be understood as a mere instrumental, referential apparatus in which signs designate or refer to objects or states of affairs, is very close to Wittgenstein's famous refutation of Augustine's conception of language. Quoting Augustine's account of his experience of language acquisition, Wittgenstein remarks, "These words, it seems to me, give us a particular picture of the essence of human language. It is this: the words in language name objects, and sentences are combinations of such names. In this picture of language we find the roots of the following idea: Every word has a meaning. This meaning is correlated with the word. It is the object for which the word stands."[10] Instead of the traditional ostensive understanding of language, Wittgenstein suggests that such a conception in fact presupposes a whole array of assumptions underlying the structural complexity of language (which he later defines in terms of "language games" and "forms of life"). According to Wittgenstein, when we say that we understand a word, we do not necessarily refer "to that which happens while we are saying or hearing it, but to the whole environment of the event of saying it."[11] Wittgenstein's similarity to Herder lies, moreover, in the idea that there is no preexistent world of objects simply present out there, ready for language to grasp and convey; rather, it is the very activity and use of language that constitute our experience for us. To put this in terms closer to Herder, language has a way of constituting the world for us by way of allowing us to pay attention to it linguistically.[12]

Herder addresses similar ideas in his "Fragments on German Literature" (1767–78) where he defines language as interdependent with thought, writing that "if it is true that we cannot think without thoughts, and learn to think through words, then language sets limits and outline for the whole of human cognition. . . . [I]t is indeed obvious that thinking is almost nothing but speaking. . . .

We think in language, whether we are explaining what is present or seeking what is not yet present" (*Fragments* 49–50). Herder then continues by arguing that each individual speaker of a language cannot but imprint his own thoughts and feelings on the very words he uses. Put differently, our words express not merely some external, independent facts but rather convey the individual way in which we, each of us uniquely, approach and, indeed, form the world in our consciousness. In "Cognition and Sensation" Herder addresses the same problem from its other end: the "medium of our self-feeling and mental consciousness," Herder writes, "is—language." In the same vein, language becomes prerequisite to what Herder calls our innermost seeing and hearing (*Cognition* 211). The resemblance to Wittgenstein is clear.

Language and Attention

Herder describes Besonnenheit in terms of attention: "The human being demonstrates [beweiset] reflection [Reflexion] when the force of his soul operates so freely that in the whole ocean of sensations [Empfindungen] which floods the soul through all the senses [der sie durch, alle Sinnen durchrauschet] it can, so to speak, separate off [absondern], stop [sie anhalten], and pay attention [Aufmerksamkeit] to a single wave" (*Treatise* 87/*AS* 722). The human being is engulfed by a powerful flood of vehement sensations that overwhelm him as they storm through (*durchrauschet*) his soul, leaving him submerged under its power (a few lines later Herder characterizes the flood as markedly less violent when he describes it in terms of a "hovering dream [schwebenden Traum] of images" that lightly touches, even caresses man).[13] Besonnenheit emanates from this scene as a force, in two respects: it is a force in its capacity to distinguish the human being from all other creatures, but it is also a force in that it bestows on man a unique strength or potency in encountering the world. Herder gives a detailed account of this process: Although he is inundated by the flood of sensations, man is able to "collect himself into a moment of alertness, freely dwell on a single image, pay it clear, more leisurely heed" [in helle, ruhigere Obacht nehmen] (*Treatise* 87/*AS* 722). Besonnenheit endows man with the ability to control and organize the world through awareness and attention, providing the conditions for introducing a distance between him and his overpoweringly immediate experience of the world. This results in a uniquely human way of experiencing the world. The importance of this argument lies in that Besonnenheit does not constitute a specific content of perception which would then somehow be translated into a linguistic expression. Here Herder suggests a view that comes close to twentieth-century ideas following the linguistic turn: Besonnenheit does not provide a content prior to language; it *is* language since for Herder, humans' perception and experience of the world is tantamount to their linguistic abilities.[14]

Herder's reflective function is crucial for the understanding not only of Besonnenheit itself but also of the very heart of his conception of language. The acquisition of language (here almost completely coeval with the capacity to reflect) inheres not simply in speech or communication. It essentially involves man's unique way of approaching the world and taking it in. Besonnenheit is not merely a capacity of paying heed to or being aware of "a single wave" or image, it is deeper than that, as the sentence continues, and has the power to "be conscious of its own attentiveness" (*Treatise* 87/*AS* 722). Besonnenheit has a dual function: first, it is the human ability to withdraw and stand back, directing attention to a single "wave" out of the totality of the flood. Second, it represents man's ability to single out, beyond the wave or image, himself as well in the very act of paying attention. Besonnenheit is, therefore, not only about the human capacity of awareness and attention, but also about man's awareness of his "own attentiveness"—that is, reflection. Herder describes a movement outward of consciousness toward the flood, a movement that stops to pay attention to its distinguishable parts: flood, objects and consciousness itself. Herder makes a point of separating between recognition of the distinct properties of the object, and acknowledgment and awareness of the mind's own operation (*Treatise* 87/*AS* 722). Man becomes aware of himself as a creature that is independent from the flood by way of his capacity of awareness and reflection: by way of being a creature of language.[15]

Having language means, therefore, that humans are able to come back to themselves and to reflect on the very act of their being aware of the world. This demonstrates why the primary language of sensations cannot be sufficient for Herder. In order to provide a proper transition between animal and human language, Herder must introduce the element of reflection which he links to the freedom inherent in human self-awareness and intention. In Herder's theory of language, animals and humans are each specifically positioned in the world through their unique capacities (linguistic or other); each can experience the world and relate to it. What distinguishes them from one another is the freedom inscribed in man's ability to reflect and thus to be in relation to himself, find himself in reflection, not by instinct: man "becomes free standing [freistehend], can seek for himself a sphere for self-mirroring, can mirror himself within himself" [kann sich in sich bespiegeln] (*Treatise* 82/*AS* 717). Von Mücke suggests that we understand this formulation (and others like it in the *Treatise*) in terms of narcissism: whereas Herder defines the animal with regard to its outside (albeit narrow) world, "man's faculties are organized and structured only in regard to themselves. In a self-reflective manner, he constitutes the totality of his otherwise diffused and disorganized faculties." Humans' center of gravity resides, therefore, in a complex combination between the inner and the outer as they appear in the mirror-relation entrenched in Herder's understanding of human reflection.[16]

Although Besonnenheit crucially includes dimensions of reflection and reason, it also comprises feeling among its constituents. Its unique awareness does not amount to a mere extraction of a "wave" or object from the flood: Herder describes it in terms of a certain quiet clarity, a calm, fixed awareness. A feeling of calm and composure accompanies the act of *Besinnung* which is thus revealed as not a merely cognitive or rational moment (*Treatise* 87/*AS* 722). Since Besonnenheit is not just added to the domain of feeling but functions as a constitutive factor, it transforms the sensory stimulus into determinate content. Hence, the system of signs does not contradict perception; rather, perception realizes itself fully only in those signs, in language.[17] And so, to solve the enigma of the transition from natural to abstract language, Herder combines perception and naming and treats them as two continuous segments of the same act: there is no separation or transition between the two phases so that signified and sign *become one and the same thing.*

Herder is very critical of those who have searched for the origin of language in the improvement of primordial instruments of articulation, in the animal sounds of passion or in the imitation of natural sounds "as though anything could be meant by such a blind inclination, and as though the ape with precisely this inclination, or the blackbird which is so good at aping sounds, had invented a language!" (*Treatise* 89/*AS* 724). But he is most fiercely opposed to those who assume that the origin of language is in mere convention or social agreement: "Here it is no *cry of sensation,* for no breathing machine but a creature taking awareness invented language! *No principle of imitation* [Nachahmung] in the soul. . . . Least of all is it *common-understanding,* arbitrary societal convention" (*Treatise* 90/*AS* 725). Herder dismisses the imitative and social origins of language; in the *Treatise,* the origin of language lies in the human capacities of reflection and attention (grounded in Besonnenheit) rather than in the ability to speak or articulate sounds, or the possibility of being understood by another: "Here it is no *organization* of the mouth which produces language, for even the person who was dumb all his life, if he was a human being, if he took awareness, had language in his soul [so lag Sprache in seiner Seele]! . . . [T]he savage, the solitary in the forest, would necessarily have invented language for himself even if he had never spoken it" [hätte er sie auch nie geredet] (*Treatise* 90/*AS* 725). Understanding language as an internal configuration of human perception and mind, Herder emphasizes its inherent detachment from speech and communication.[18] Herder does not dismiss the acoustic elements of language altogether, yet he foregrounds the dissociation between these elements and the *origin* of language. Even if humans eventually come to speak their language and use it as a means of communication, language's origin or its essence do not lie there. Herder establishes this radical argument by bringing the human soul into the discussion. This provides the basis for his alternative explanation.

From its first appearance in the text, Besonnenheit is linked to the human soul and defined as a "force of his soul" (*Kraft seiner Seele*) (*Treatise* 87/*AS* 722). The capacity to stand back and pay attention, the ability to distinguish one wave from within the overwhelming flood, and finally, the human faculty of reflection—are all operations of the soul: "where *concepts intersect* and *get entangled*!, where the *most diverse feelings produce* one another [einander erzeugen], where a *pressing occasion summons forth all the forces of the soul* and *reveals the whole art of invention of which the soul is capable*" (*Treatise* 115/*AS* 754).[19]

Though Herder is deeply concerned with the senses and sense perception (as I will discuss in detail) even when he discusses the three central senses (sight, touch, and hearing), the human soul still features as his core notion. Besonnenheit allows man to be open to the world and the world to inscribe itself his soul: "Even if his mouth and his eye remained forever closed, his soul does not remain entirely without language . . . without eyes and tongue, to *name* them in his soul" (*Treatise* 98–99/*AS* 735). The human soul, however, not only conditions humans' openness to their surroundings: more important, it accommodates their reflective faculty. Herder writes accordingly that "language was the common-understanding of his soul with itself [Einverständnis seiner Seele mit sich], and a common-understanding as necessary as the human being was human being" [als der Mensch Mensch war] (*Treatise* 90/*AS* 725). The reflective constituent of language inherent to Besonnenheit manifests itself when the soul stands in relation to itself, reflecting upon itself in, as Herder puts it, *Einverständnis*. This German term signifies something more than mere common understanding, as the English translation of the *Treatise* puts it, referring, in addition, to an internal accord or unison between man and his soul, and between the soul and itself. This internal, reflective accord is essential to the human being's being human.[20]

"You Are the Bleating One": Language and Sound

Herder illustrates the workings of Besonnenheit and with it, the formation of reflective human language, by way of an elaborate (and renowned) example: that of the bleating sheep (he initially uses "a lamb" [*jenes Lamm*], and then continues with "sheep" [*Schaf*]). Herder is not the first to use this example. Moses Mendelssohn used it more than twenty years earlier (1756), in a letter to Lessing written just after he finished translating Rousseau's "Second Discourse."[21] As Von Mücke points out, Mendelssohn's letter attempts to "save"

Rousseau from some of the problematic aspects of his own essay by showing that although he seemingly praises savage man over social man, Rousseau in fact harbors a much more positive attitude toward human society. The sheep appears as part of Mendelssohn's explanation of the development from a natural to a social state, serving to demonstrate how man learns to associate between images and sounds.[22] Although the sheep proves to be an excellent way into his argument, Herder's choice raises a question: why is it that he chooses a domesticated animal, an animal that is potentially, at least, humanized? We could say that there is a potential "impurity" in this choice, especially because the sound of the bleating is translatable into a human utterance: Ah, Bha, and so on. Johann Georg Hamann picks this up in his interesting discussions of Herder's *Treatise*, especially *The Last Will and Testament of the Knight of the Rose-Cross* and *Philological Ideas and Doubts*, and *To the Solomon of Prussia*.[23] I will present Herder's example of the sheep in detail, since it not only bears on my previous arguments but also brings out the central role of sound and hearing in his theory of language. In order to substantiate the specifically human character of Besonnenheit, Herder introduces his account of the sheep from a dual perspective: the animal and human. This is how he stages the scene: a sheep appears—but it appears in an entirely different manner before the eyes of animals and those of men.

While it is specifically the human being, and not the animal, who is overwhelmed by the flood of sensations, the animal too is taken over, not by sensation as such, but by its own instincts. The "hungry, scenting wolf" or "the blood-licking lion" are overpowered by their instincts (Herder writes that "sensuality has overcome them" [Sinnlichkeit hat sie überwältigt] [*Treatise* 88/*AS* 723]) which causes them to see or smell nothing but the sheep's flesh, impelling them to attack it. The "aroused ram" too, is guided by his sensuality and instinct, perceiving the female sheep only as a potential object of sexual pleasure. Other animals whose instincts direct them toward a different focal point, are completely indifferent (*gleichgültig*) to the sheep as it passes by them almost unnoticed. Herder uses the terms "light" and "shade" here, emphasizing the sharp contrast between the indifferent animal that allows the sheep to pass by in light-dark shades (*klar-dunkel vorbeistreichen läßt*), and the intense directedness of instinct that as it were casts a narrow, focused light beam on its object, not allowing the instinctively driven animal to notice anything else outside this narrow span: it is in this sense that the lion, for instance, does not see the sheep as a whole, but only its edible flesh, whereas the ant passes completely indifferent to either the lion's or the sheep's existence.[24] This echoes, of course, the previous discussion of the animal's "circles of life" and the sharp and distinct, yet narrow and limited, perspective from which it experiences, or finds itself in, the world (*Treatise* 78–81/*AS* 712–715).

A human being is not impelled by animal instincts, nor is he indifferent toward the lamb: "Let that lamb pass before his eye," Herder writes, "as an image [als Bild]—[something that happens] to him as to no other animal" (*Treatise* 88/*AS* 723). Herder's use of "image" emphasizes the middle position that human beings occupy—not too close yet not too far—exactly between the indomitable power of instinct and cold, detached indifference. Man is not governed by his instincts, Herder explains, and this is precisely what allows him to grasp the sheep as a whole, and eventually, as an object (this would be categorically different from the forceful, yet partial, perception possible in the case of the lion or ram). In perceiving the lamb as image, man occupies a perfect distance: he neither needs it nor is he indifferent to it (Herder's use of "image" here is interesting, since as the argument continues, his account steers clear from vision, accentuating instead the sense of hearing). This middle position of man, not too close yet not too far, implies a uniquely human desire to know the object: "As soon as he [man] develops a need [Bedürfnis] to become acquainted with the sheep, no instinct disturbs him, no sense tears him too close to the sheep or away from it" [so störet ihm kein Instinkt: so reißt ihn kein Sinn auf dasselbe zu nahe hin oder davon ab] (*Treatise* 88/*AS* 723).[25]

It is also worthwhile at this point to return to Mendelssohn's interesting use of the same example. In his account of Rousseau's natural state, Mendelssohn describes a "savage" encountering a sheep that stands in a flowery meadow. Upon hearing the sound of the bleating, the savage can perceive it as belonging to the sheep, but he can also associate it with the entire setting (the meadow, flowers, as well as the sheep). This demonstrates, Mendelssohn argues, how natural sounds can be transformed into arbitrary signs.[26] In the *Treatise,* as we have begun to see, Herder takes a different line of argument.

Since it is now not merely a tasty piece of flesh (to the lion) or a means for sexual satisfaction (for the ram), the sheep can stand before man "exactly as it expresses itself to his senses" (*Treatise* 88/*AS* 723). It stands as it is in its wholeness, and more important, as it expresses itself, and not as a mirror of man's own instinctive "light beams."[27] Man is receptive to the world, open to it, and the sheep is now active before him: it expresses itself rather than being a mere fulfillment of another creature's need. The sheep does not pass before man's eyes (or ears) as an object satisfying a need or instinct, yet the description of its appearance is extremely palpable and sensuous. It is almost as if Herder renders man's way of perceiving the sheep in its every detail, but in so doing in fact, projects himself as confronting the sheep.

This is a crucial point in the argument, as Herder addresses the distinctive way in which Besonnenheit approaches the sheep. Merely locating the human being as not too close yet not too far does not suffice. Herder must give an account of the human language, defined by awareness and reflection, rather than the immediacy of instinct. How exactly is the human being aware of the sheep, and in what sense is this awareness linguistic? Man needs to recognize what Herder calls a characteristic-mark (*Merkmal*), which distinguishes the sheep qua sheep, separating it like a wave from the all-encompassing flood of perceptions and sensations. Herder will eventually indicate that this characteristic mark is the origin of the first word; but this word is unrelated to any human utterance, imitation of sound or expression: it is an internally imprinted mark, an inner word in man's soul. Owing to the capacity of Besonnenheit, the soul recognizes the sheep "in a human way," and man is able to turn the characteristic mark into an internal name of the sheep, imprinting it on his soul. What would this characteristic mark be, given humans have no instinct guiding them toward it? It is not the sheep's white color, nor is it its soft wool or distinct size. The human soul finds the characteristic mark in the sheep's bleating—in the sound that it makes, and with the bleating, "the inner sense takes effect" [Der innere Sinn würket] (*Treatise* 88/*AS* 723).

It is evident that bleating is a sound distinctive to the sheep, a sound no other creature produces in quite the same way. But Herder argues that bleating is not merely an example but an exemplar, in that sound is primary here: sound in general and not only that of the sheep. Sound takes a primary role in the human perception of the sheep and the eventual formation of a characteristic mark. Sound, Herder argues, makes the strongest impression on the human soul. The sound quality of the bleating therefore enables it to be torn away (*losriß*) from the sheep as an enclosed (white, soft, woolly) object, leaping forth and making its way directly into the confines of the human soul. Herder uses the word *eindrängen* (penetrate) here, to communicate the violent, irresistible force with which the sound of bleating enters the soul. Neither the sight nor the touch of the sheep has a comparable impact, as only sound can actively move from the object toward the human soul and enter it.[28]

This unique capacity of sound to penetrate the soul emerges on man's first encounter with the sheep. But it reappears, and more forcefully, on the second encounter: the soul recognizes the bleating and makes it into the distinguishing feature of the sheep. This time, however, the bleating is not only seared into the soul but is named with a characteristic mark (*Treatise* 88/*AS* 723). Herder situates language within the soul rather than conceiving it as operating vis-à-vis the external world of perceived sense data, and in doing so he accentuates the complex relations between internal and external, perception and expression, human and world. Although his argument is couched in terms of reflection (the soul "speaking to itself"), Herder provides us with a complex case that challenges the sharp demarcation between inside and outside.

It is important to dwell on this moment of recognition, since it is a key to the understanding of the movement from Besonnenheit as a form of perception, to its function as language. Besonnenheit opens the human being to the world, enabling him to be struck by it, be astonished by the force of its imprint on his soul. This occurs, in Herder's account, through the unique way in which man pays attention. This attentiveness enables man to identify the sheep as separate and distinct in the flood of perceptions, but it allows him a further and crucial step. The human being is able to re-encounter the sheep and experience it as a unified entity: "you are the bleating *one*." Not only does the bleating penetrate the soul and reveal a characteristic mark of the sheep, but everything that has to do with the sheep is now united around it, and the sheep as "one" crystallizes around its acoustic core. Here the component of awareness and reflection emerges and eventually allows the movement from the indistinct zone of Besonnenheit to the more properly human specificity of *Besinnung*, from the flood of sensations to a name.[29]

This is why Herder chooses to focus on the human soul here rather than on perception or even abstract thought. The soul is the space into which the "raw" perceptual data flow from the outside and is arranged together and become unified and attributed to the sheep. The characteristic mark of the sheep, its bleating, becomes its name for the soul. This is an eminently linguistic moment, where human Besonnenheit finally appears as the very thing Herder is looking for, namely, the origin of language: "This *first characteristic mark of taking-awareness* [Besinnung] *was a word of the soul* [Wort der Seele]*! With it human language is invented*" (*Treatise* 88/*AS* 723). Herder's "word of the soul" appears several times in the *Treatise* as the first and essential condition of language. Since the human being is defined as a linguistic creature, it follows that every perception, feeling or thought, also has an inherently linguistic structure: there is "*no condition in the human soul which does not turn out to be susceptible of words or actually determined by words of the soul*."[30]

Herder notes that this internal word is not spoken or acoustically expressed, nor does it need to be communicated to or understood by others; it is imprinted and reverberates internally: "even if the human being's tongue had never tried to stammer it" [nie seine Zunge zu stammeln versucht hätte] and even if he "never reached the situation of conveying this idea [diese Idee zu geben] to another creature . . . still his soul has, so to speak, bleated internally" [in ihrem Inwendigen geblökt] (*Treatise* 89/*AS* 724). In a fragment entitled "On the capacity to speak and hear" [Über die Fähigkeit zu sprechen und zu hören] (1795), Herder discusses communication in language, referring to it not as verbal or sonic communication. Rather, it is a communication between souls: "Sprache ist das Band der Seelen" [language is the bond between souls].[31] A few pages later Herder returns to a similar scene, when he describes man as "the learning child-without-any-say," or in German, *Unmündige*. Aside from its literal meaning (mouth-less), the word Unmündige carrieslegal connotations associated with those who (for instance, due to their being minors) are not allowed to speak in the courtroom, that is, their speech is prevented. In Herder's understanding of language, the Unmündige actually does speak, but it is the human soul that speaks, and to no one else but itself. In this moment, the external bleating of the sheep comes together with the internal bleating of the soul (awareness of the world and the soul's reflection upon itself), and the bleating "rang out! [es klang!] The soul laid hold [haschte]—and there it has a *resounding word*!" [tönendes Wort!] (*Treatise* 98/*AS* 734).

Herder's use of "resounding" here deserves some attention. The echo played an explicit and central role in the first pages of the *Treatise*. As I discussed in the previous chapter, Herder makes a point of describing the primary language of sensations as a language not only of immediate expression. It also elicits an immediate sympathetic response which he describes repeatedly in terms of echo: the "struck string" of animal feeling is immediately expressed and thereby "performs its natural duty [Naturpflicht]: it sounds! it calls to a similarly feeling Echo—even when none is there, even when it does not hope or expect to be answered by one" (*Treatise* 66/*AS* 697–698). Herder continues with his third formulation of the "law of nature" which becomes a "blessing" when the cry of a single, suffering creature draws an immediate response from nature in the form of an echo.[32] This is Herder's way of achieving the transformation of the mere mechanical and natural into a moral structure in which the crying animal feels part of nature as its cry echoes, or re-sounds, the response of the whole of nature back to it. Although the *Treatise*'s second section and with it, distinctly human language, has a strong basis in sound and especially hearing, the echo seems to play no role in it. However, despite Herder's argument that speech is not essential for human language, the echo is decidedly present also in the emergence of the human language of Besonnenheit.

The manifestation of echo in the second section of the *Treatise* is independent of speech or the production of sound but must be conceived, rather, in terms of repetition, agreement, and something that is reflected back. Echo is thus much more about a reflective movement within an enclosed space than merely about the repetition of sound. The origin of Herder's human language remains bound up with the echo in three senses. It emerges when man encounters the sheep and hears its bleating for the first time. An acoustic space arises between the sheep and the human ear, a space in which the sound of bleating echoes and resounds. Another reference to the echo appears when Herder describes the enclosed, reflective realm of the human soul in which the soul encounters and mirrors itself. Herder treats the reflective element in terms of an echo resounding. The third instance of echo occurs in the dual moment of bleating: the external bleating of the sheep and the internal bleating of the soul. This exemplifies the complexity of Herder's use of the echo structure: the internal bleating of the soul is neither an imitation of the external sound nor a simple, mechanical repetition. The soul's ability to echo internally establishes Herder's argument that language occurs in the soul, not in the mouth or on the tongue. Reflective human language retains the component of echo so dominant in the language of sensations, but it uncouples the echo from the physical cry or howl of pain, rendering it linguistic in a purely human sense. Language resounds in the very act of reflection and the human soul becomes its echo chamber.

It is clear by now that Herder distances himself from any understanding of language to which speech, especially of a propositional or communicative nature, is essential. But before we delve deeper into the central role for language of the ear and the sense of hearing, it is worth paying attention to two, perhaps marginal but nevertheless interesting, other forms of expression related to the mouth rather than the ear. The first is song, the second breath. In the *Treatise*, Herder argues for an essential connection between human language and animal expression, and he takes the case of *song* as the crux of his argument:

> So if the first human language was song, it was song which was as natural to the human being, as appropriate to his organs and natural drives, as the nightingale's song was natural to the nightingale . . . *Condillac, Rousseau,* and others were half on the right track here in that they derive the meter and song of the oldest languages from the cry of sensation—and without doubt sensation did indeed enliven the first sounds and elevate them. But since from the mere sounds of sensation human language could never have arisen, though this song certainly was such a language, something more is still needed in order to produce this song—and that was precisely the naming of each creature in accordance with its own language [Namennennung eines jeden Geschöpfs nach seiner Sprache]. So there sang and resounded [tönte] the whole of nature as an example, and the human being's song was a concerto of all these voices [ein Konzert aller dieser Stimmen], to the extent that his understanding needed them [sofern sie sein Verstand brauche], his sensation grasped them, his organs were able to express them. Song was born, but neither a nightingale's song nor *Leibniz's* musical language nor a mere animal's cry of sensation: an expression of the language of all creatures within the natural scale [natürlichen Tonleiter] of the human voice! (*Treatise* 104/*AS* 741–742)

Although according to Herder the human being cannot learn to sing by the mere imitation of animal voices, human language is, nevertheless, closely related to animal voices, but in a wholly different way: "As little as the nightingale sings in order to sing as an example for human beings, the way people imagine, just as little will the human being ever want to invent language for himself by trilling in imitation of the nightingale" (*Treatise* 104/*AS* 741). Here Herder calls to mind the biblical scene of Adam's original act of naming, where he names each animal according to its own voice. But Herder's interest is not in the dominion and sovereignty evident in the biblical story where man, in the act of naming, is crowned as nature's ruler. Rather, he addresses the musical character of the scene. Let me refer to David Wellbery's reading of this passage. He calls attention to two important aspects of Herder's argument about song: first, the human voice is not simply another version of the animal voice, but a unique human capacity that is not only inseparable from rationality or sensibility but constitutes the medium in which they are realized. The human voice "is an autonomous instance," Wellbery writes, "it introduces into the world an expressive *novum* that obeys its own inner dynamic and exhibits its own unique productivity."[33] Second, although the human voice is but one voice in the chorus of nature, Herder stresses its unique ability to translate and thus transpose all of nature's sounds into man's unique tonality. This is what Herder refers to here as the "concerto of all these voices." Predominant in Herder's description is the way in which the acoustic dimension subsumes everything that is human: "Everything the human being sees, feels, smells, and tastes has an inwardly audible tonal correlate, which in turn can be transformed into a voiced expression."[34] This "voiced expression" does not amount to any form of propositional speech, nor is it related to communication. The "concerto" is a sound event in which the whole of nature partakes via its expression in the human voice. The human being, in other words, does not speak (or for that matter, sing) *about* nature; he expresses it immediately in song. This description is interesting in the specific context of the relationship between human and nature; but its implications regarding human language broadly speaking are no less thought provoking.

The second type of oral expression that does not amount to speech is the case of the breath. A far more intricate account concerning breath appears in the *Ideas of a Philosophy of the History of Man* [Ideen zur Philosophie der Geschichte der Menschheit] (1784–91).[35] In his *Ideas,* Herder construes an essential connection between hearing and what he calls "a breath of air," the breath marking the nexus of man's speech, song and moan. "All that man has ever thought, willed, done, or will do upon Earth," he writes, "has depended on the movement of a breath of air, for if this divine breath had not inspired us and floated like a charm on our lips, we should all have still been wanderers in the woods" (*Ideas,* Book 9 199). The breath of air links speech and hearing, which Herder takes to be inseparable, and it operates similarly to the conjuncture between body and mind. In both cases, we can only *feel* the connection, but never comprehend the details of its operation. Everything the human being feels (Herder particularly mentions grief and joy), says and perceives, becomes *sound,* so that

> what is heard by the ear moves the tongue; that images and sensations may become mental characters, and these characters significant, nay impressive, sounds, arises from a concent[36] of so many dispositions, like a voluntary league, which the creator has thought proper to establish between the most opposite senses and instincts, powers and members, of his creature, in a manner not less wonderful than that in which the mind and body are conjoined. (*Ideas*, Book 9 199)

This account of *concent* comes very close to Herder's aforementioned description of human song as a "concerto" of all natural sounds and voices. The breath here, however, is not only a song or concerto, but also an image: "The breath of our mouth is the picture of the world" (*Ideas*, Book 9 232). The breath is the human way of expressing a relation to the world, by painting its picture, but not through an act of representation or of referentially pointing at it. The human being relates to the world by way of his and her mere breath.[37]

Interestingly, it is the above sentence from *Ideas* that Heidegger chooses to quote in his "What Are Poets For?"[38] in the context of his discussion of language, song, and poetry. Although I discuss Heidegger's relationship to Herder's thought in detail in chapter 4, a few words are called for here. Without considering for the moment on Heidegger's important account of poetic language in this essay, it is useful to explore his unique reference to Herder at this point and glance at the way in which Herder's thought affected Heidegger's later philosophy. Toward the end of his essay Heidegger quotes Herder in the context of his own interpretation of Rilke's *Sonnets to Orpheus*, just after his discussion of the difference between a concept of language as making propositional assertions and what he calls language as "saying." Bringing together Rilke's sonnets and Herder's *Ideas*, Heidegger contends that the breath is nothing less than the very nature of language. At the end of the third sonnet Rilke writes: "To sing in truth is another breath [In Wahrheit singen, ist ein andrer Hauch]. A breath for nothing [Ein Hauch um nichts] . . . A wind."[39] Those who "dare," or "the more venturesome" ones in Heidegger's account, are daring by virtue of their very breath, which does not ask or reach for "this or that objective thing." The breath of those who dare is therefore, "a breath for nothing." Heidegger suggests here a surprising link between Herder's two aforementioned accounts of song and breath. "The singer's saying says the sound whole of worldly existence, which invisibly offers its space within the world's inner space of the heart. The song does not even first follow what is to be said. . . . Song itself is 'a wind.' "[40] Singing turns away from propositional speech of assertions and does not solicit a production of anything. "In the song," Heidegger continues, "the world's inner space concedes space within itself."[41] Song and breath come together in Heidegger's reading of Rilke's sonnet and appear as the two extremes of speechless, yet expressive, language in Herder.

An Ear for Language

Herder devotes a lengthy discussion to the sense of hearing, comparing it to sight and touch (*Gefühl*) (I use "touch" rather than "sense" here to reserve the latter word for Herder's comparison between the three *senses*), so as to establish hearing's primacy over the other senses as well as its being what Herder calls the only "sense of language." After establishing the central role of hearing in the development of human language, Herder seeks to establish that hearing is the only "sense of language" by way of a detailed comparison between the sense of hearing on the one hand, and sight and touch on the other.[42] Herder presents this comparison in terms of six features: distance, distinctness and clarity, relationship between human and world, temporal structure, the need to express, and humans' physical/biological development. For each feature, he presents a detailed comparison between the three senses—and in each case, he reaches the conclusion that hearing is the "middle sense," not too cold and far (like vision) and not too close (like touch). The sense of hearing is precisely in the middle, thereby connecting between the different senses, forming perception into language.

Herder begins with an account of the "sphere of sensibility from outside," to which the sense of touch brings us too close (sensing everything only in itself), whereas the sense of vision opens too large a distance (taking us too far out of ourselves). Being placed exactly in the middle, the sense of hearing positions the human being precisely at the right distance from the world so as to be able to take it in, unite it into a single, distinct experience that, in turn, becomes language: "We become, so to speak, hearing through all our senses! . . . [W]hat one sees, what one feels, becomes soundable as well. The sense for language has become our middle and unifying sense; we are linguistic creatures" [Sprachgeschöpfe] (*Treatise* 109/*AS* 747). The second argument in his comparison of the senses refers to the "distinctness and clarity" of perception. Touch is too obscure, whereas sight is too clear—both senses are unfit to supply man with the necessary capacities to distinguish the wave from the flood, or bleating as the sheep's characteristic mark. In this case too, hearing is the sense that brings it all together, clarifying what is too obscure, and unifying the dispersed, "and since this acknowledgment of the manifold through one, through a characteristic mark, becomes language, hearing is language" [or, in the first version of the *Treatise*: the organ of language: *Organ der Sprache*] (*Treatise* 110/*AS* 748).

Skipping the third proposition, which I discuss in more detail later in this chapter, Herder's fourth characteristic of hearing relates to its temporal form. With both the sense of touch and sight we take everything in at once, touch stirring "our strings strongly but briefly and in jumps," and vision intimidating our pupils, "through the immeasurable canvas of its *side-by-side*." In hearing, on the other hand, nature "counts sounds into our souls only one after another, gives and never tires, gives and always has more to give. . . [S]he [nature] *teaches progressively!* Who in these circumstances could not grasp language, invent language for himself?" (*Treatise* 110/*AS* 748–749). Hearing is the only sense through which, Herder claims, the soul can experience the sequence of impressions, its flow that can only be experienced in time.[43]

The following, fifth proposition accounts for hearing's unique correspondence to the human need to express itself. When touching, humans are concerned only with themselves; they are "selfish and self-engrossed"; vision is inexpressible since the viewed object remains before the eye even if it is never expressed. The objects of hearing, conversely, are connected with movement and thereby must resound: "They become expressible because they must be expressed, and . . . through their movement, do they become expressible." As Forester notes, Herder's use of "because" here denotes a need or purpose, whereas "through" refers to the enabling conditions of means of expressions.[44] We are again faced with hearing's distinguished status as the sense for language.

Finally, hearing is also the middle sense in terms of humans' physical development. Although touch is the first sense operative in the embryo, it is only through hearing that these first sensations can unfold, "since nature awakens the soul to its first distinct sensation through sounds . . . awakens it out of the obscure sleep of *feeling* and ripens it to still finer sensuality." Hearing is where touch and vision cooperate, since the human being "took the path from feeling into the sense of his visual images [Phantasmen] no otherwise than via the sense of language, and has hence learned to sound forth what he sees as much as what he felt" (*Treatise* 111/*AS* 750).[45]

Let me go back now to Herder's third proposition about the sense of hearing. Herder's comparison here is between the ways in which the world thrusts itself onto the human soul via the three senses at stake. The sense of touch has an overpowering quality (*überwältigen*) due to which the outside world almost attacks the sensitive human soul, penetrating it too forcefully. The sense of sight, on the other hand, has a cold and distant quality, which renders man somewhat indifferent to what he experiences as it remains "too much at rest before us." These two possibilities put the human being at a remove from his linguistic nature. Hearing, once more, figures as the "middle" way: "we can for longer and almost for ever hear, think words with hearing, so to speak; hearing is for the soul what green, the middle color, is for sight" (*Treatise* 110/*AS* 748). When man hears he is not overwhelmed, but neither does he remain indifferent. When man hears its bleating, the sheep comes to matter to him—not because of its meat or wool but because the sound of its bleating has entered his soul. This idea is interestingly echoed in Herder's remarks on sound in *Fourth Grove*. There he speaks of what he calls the "inwardness of hearing." Comparing between the senses, he situates touch, vision, and hearing in the intermediate between external and internal. Touch marks the physical perimeter of our bodies and is therefore the most "external" of the three senses. As for vision, although I perceive the visual image of an external object through the eye and it is, as it were, taken in, the object of that image remains external to me. A sound, on the other hand, is not inseparable from the object that produced it and can thereby come closer to our interior, the ear being closest to the soul. Nature acknowledges this, Herder continues, "for she knew no better path to the soul than through the ear and through language."[46] The sound of the bleating tears itself away from the animal that originally produced it, so that it achieves independence and moves toward the human ear. Hanly writes in this context that Herder uses the sheep's bleating as a paradigm constituting the origin of the first word in sounding, thereby turning listening not merely into a conceptual starting point but rather into the very "nexus around which the entire possibility of the human will gather[s] and coalesce[s]. Besinnung, in this sense, *is* precisely a listening."[47]

In the first pages of the *Treatise*, when Herder speaks of sympathy and the cry of pain, he discusses what is commonly addressed in the eighteenth century as the problem of "sense deprivation," specifically the case of blindness. Herder argues with Diderot's claim that since the visual scene of suffering and pain is shrouded for those who are born blind, they are doomed to be less sensitive to it than those who see. According to Herder, the opposite is the case: "There he listens in darkness, consequently, in the stillness of his eternal night, and each moan penetrates his heart that much more deeply and sharply, like an arrow!" (*Treatise* 73/*AS* 706). The encounter with the pain of another visually as well as acoustically is too intrusive and overwhelming for the human soul. The deprivation of sight in the case of the blind suggests an alternative in which the sense of hearing, divested of all visual distractions, becomes more attentive, acute, and penetrating. Hearing the painful cry, rather than seeing the entire scene, emerges as the condition of possibility for genuine, deep human sympathy. Herder ends by adding the sense of touch to the blind person who when touching the shaking, suffering body, makes it entirely his own, feels the other's pain as it "shoots through" his own body as well as his "inner nerve structure," producing a deep sense of sympathy (*Treatise* 73/*AS* 706).

Another version of this argument in the *Ideas* is the example of those born deaf and dumb. Herder explains, that lacking the ability to hear and speak, they cannot accomplish their potential of human reason, and more crucially, they are unable to distinguish between their own human species and other animal species. "We have more than one instance," he writes, "of a person born deaf and dumb, who murdered his brother in consequence of having seen a pig killed, and tore out his bowels with tranquil pleasure" (*Ideas*, Book 9 87). Herder's very specific emphasis here is thought provoking if not problematic: the absence of hearing and speech in the deaf and dumb generates not only violent behavior, but more importantly, an inability to empathize with the suffering of members of their own species.

Another reason that hearing is crucial for Herder is that it is the only sense capable of transforming sonic sense data into words, thus becoming the original sense of, and for, language. Herder dwells on sound's uniquely intimate capacity of penetrating the human soul so that "it inevitably becomes a characteristic mark, but still not so stunningly that it could not become a clear characteristic mark" [Der Ton des Gehörs dringt so innig in unsre Seele, daß er Merkmal werden muß; aber noch nicht so übertäubend, daß er nicht klares Merkmal werden könnte]. The sense of hearing enables sounds to penetrate the soul and take hold of it, without violating or impinging on it; in Trabant's words: "Hearing is an unviolent sublimated form of erotic touch."[48] This erotic "intimacy" that Herder describes here is a specific form of closeness which, while not threatening or intrusive, nevertheless creates a shared space of kinship. Within this space sound becomes, or rather, must become, a *clear* characteristic mark (and not a mere characteristic mark). The sheep's bleating can become an internal bleating of the soul, which in turn, is the very beginning of language: hearing is therefore "the sense for language" (*Treatise* 110/*AS* 748).

Ah! and Aha!

The question of the kinship between Herder's original, primary language of sensations and reflective human language reopens when one considers the central role of hearing in both. Trabant discusses what he calls Herder's rediscovery of the ear for language philosophy in terms of a philosophical revolution:[49] "If it is language which makes man human, and if the ear is the organ of that human thing, then the ear is the human sense par excellence. . . . [T]he ear is—no matter what Derrida says—the most important organ for the humanization of man."[50] Herder's striking claim that human language exists independently of speech or communication does not dissociate his theory of language from sound altogether. Quite the contrary, as both the primary language of sensations and reflective language include a crucial sonic element. In the language of sensations, this element is Philoctetes' cry of pain or what Herder describes later in the text as the exclamation "Ah!"; in the case of human language, the sheep's bleating captures man's attention and triggers the process of linguistic attention and reflection, leading man to the "Aha!" of recognition. In both cases, however, the origin, essence, and development of language are determined not by the capacity to produce sound, but rather by the ability to hear it; or more boldly put: by the inability not to hear it. But before I present Herder's arguments about the sense of hearing and its inherent kinship with language, I would like to dwell on what I take to be the essential relationship between the emergence of sound in Herder's linguistic theory and the problem of pain.

In the first part of the *Treatise*, the cry of pain is deemed fundamental insofar as it elicits an immediate sympathetic feeling in all of nature. This shared feeling, which serves as the ground of the language of sensations, is not determined by any specific content communicated by the suffering man or animal but by the very act of expressing it. The pained "Ah!" immediately penetrates and moves all other creatures, drawing them into a form of participation. When Herder asks "Who is there who, faced with a shaking, whining tortured person, with a moaning dying person, and even with a groaning farm animal when its whole machine is suffering, is not touched to his heart by this 'Ah!'?" [dies Ach nicht zu Herzen dringe?], rather than posing a moral problem, this rhetorical question describes the natural state of the language of sensations. The sound of pain creates and assembles the linguistic community around it so that "they really share each other's pain mechanically" (*Treatise* 72/*AS* 705–706). The intensity of pain's expression undermines the enclosed singularity of every individual (man and animal), bringing them together in what Herder would understand as nothing less than language.[51]

Despite Herder's insistence on the categorical separation between the language of sensation and language of reflection in the two parts of the *Treatise*, both figure in a surprisingly similar manner if we consider the sense of hearing. Human language is formed on the basis of Besonnenheit's capacity to call man's attention from the flood of sensations. Separating the sheep's bleating from all other sense data becomes therefore the condition under which alone the first word is formed: "But listen! [Aber horch!] The sheep bleats! There a characteristic mark of itself tears itself free from the canvas of the color picture in which so little could be distinguished" (*Treatise* 98/*AS* 735). When man encounters the sheep for the second time, he recognizes it: " 'Aha! You are the bleating one!' [du bist das Blökende!] the soul feels inwardly" [fühlt sie innerlich] (*Treatise* 88/*AS* 723).[52] In addition to the bleating here the "Aha!" associated with the soul's recognition of the sheep's characteristic mark plays a crucial role. In the context of his linguistic abilities, the world appears before the human being neither in visual images, nor by way of touch; it appears in sounds, cries, hisses.

Herder's emphasis on sound is significant not only as the sense through which the world appears and is experienced but because sound, specifically, has the power to penetrate the human soul: "Nature herself," he writes in *Fourth Grove*, "knew no better path to the soul than through the ear and through language" (250). Sound constitutes a space within which the human encounters the world: the bleating "has penetrated deeply and distinctly into the soul [in die

Seele gedrungen]. "Aha!" . . . now I will know you again. You bleat!" . . . Reason [Vernunft] and language took a timid step together, and nature came to meet them half-way *through hearing*. Nature sounded the characteristic mark not only forth but deep into the soul!" (*Treatise* 98/*AS* 734). Perceiving the world, the human being is situated *in it* rather than facing it. Humans are in accord with the world via a profound sense of taking part in it—by means of their ability to hear it, listen to it. The ear becomes the center of the universe, so to speak, holding it together, harmonizing it.

The emphasis here is on the fact that the sound of bleating is not only voiced "forth" but also reaches "deep" into the soul—and this is precisely what distinguishes sound for Herder: its unique capacity to move forth from its original object and penetrate another, becoming an integral part of it. The sense of hearing plays a dual role for Herder: first, through hearing the world seems to speak to man, to address him in sounds. Second, the sense of hearing creates an internal linguistic space in which humans appear before themselves as beings-in-the-world. Instead of appearing an external, foreign entity confronted by the human, the world, through hearing, appears as an integral part of the human soul, it appears *for* human beings. In the intersection between these two functions, the "Ah!" of the language of sensations comes together with the "Aha!" of Besonnenheit and human language. In both cases there is a decisive sonic element: the immediate cry of pain that evokes primary natural sympathy which is the characteristic mark of the language of sensations: Ah! and on the other hand, the sound of bleating which the human soul recognizes and makes into a characteristic mark, a word of the soul: "Aha!"

The relationship between the Ah! of the *Treatise*'s first section and the Aha! of the second, gains an interesting perspective when we compare the role of the sheep in the *Treatise* to its altogether different appearance in Herder's *Ideas*. Whereas in the *Treatise*, Herder makes a point of distancing humans' way of relating to the sheep from that of the instinctive animal that relates to the sheep solely in terms of its needs, in *Ideas*, the human's attitude to the sheep (representing animals in general) is thoroughly instrumental. Herder describes the human being as

> benefiting himself by such [animals] as were useful, and rendering himself the general lord of every thing in nature: for in every one of his appropriations he does nothing in reality but mark the character of a tameable, useful being, to be employed for his own convenience. . . . In the gentle sheep, for instance, he remarked the milk sucked by the lamb, and the wool that warmed his hand, and endeavored to appropriate each to his own use. (*Ideas*, Book 9 240)

This is a very different account from that in the *Treatise*. The sheep appears before the human being only insofar as it is useful to the latter, and the human being indeed appropriates, in Herder's words, the sheep—or for that matter, any other animal or natural object. In the *Ideas*, the human closely resembles the blood-licking lion or the aroused ram, overcome by their instinct and sensuality, impelled to attack the sheep (*Treatise* 88/*AS* 723). Although in both texts, the sheep exemplifies something about the origin of the human relationship to the environment, these texts give a very different account of this relationship. In *Ideas*, man experiences the sheep in terms of the potential satisfaction of his needs, an approach that comes to be the definition of his situatedness in the world. In the *Treatise*, on the other hand, the sheep is precisely *not* conceived in relation to need: here it is the fact of its being situated at the right distance, according to Herder, neither too far nor too close, that matters: a distance permitting calm, collected reflection.

Kelly Oliver uses the above quoted passage from the *Ideas* as a basis for a critique of Herder's choice to refer to an abstract, generalized animal which he can thus approach from a functional point of view. Considering specific animals (or, for that matter, human beings) would have enabled further variation and continuity in the account of human-animal relations. Oliver continues with a fierce critique of what she identifies as Herder's blind spot, namely, the fact that despite his insistence on humans' godlike superiority over animals, in fact he completely depends on them for the constitution of their own language: "Man's unique capacity for understanding, knowing, reason, transcending instinct, emulation, speech, differentiation, observation, recognition, recollection, and ownership—everything that defines man as man and as human—comes through an encounter with the sheep."[53] Herder's use of the animal as an example, in other words, comes to deal with the threat the animal poses to the human's alleged autonomy. While Oliver's criticism may be justified in the context of her overall concern, namely, the importance of animals in how we learn to be human, in the context of Herder's argument in the *Treatise*, her interpretation can be somewhat misguiding. Let me try to offer a different explanation of the role of the animal in Herder's conception of language.

Since I take the *Treatise*'s first two sections *not* to be mutually exclusive, though this is how Herder himself presents it in the *Treatise*, I would like here to demonstrate how primordial animal-human language remains closely intimate with distinctly human, reflective language. The appearance of the sheep in the account of human language is crucial in this respect. Herder presents the sheep, from the outset, to elucidate his broader claim regarding human language and, in many respects, the human being as such. And yet it is no mere example. Herder's choice to locate the origin of human language in the human's encounter with an animal rather than with another human being is significant, first, since it underlines that for Herder human language does not originate from the need to communicate or as part of any other form of intersubjectivity. Foregrounding the encounter with an animal is all the more significant by providing Herder with a way of not altogether abandoning the primordial language of immediate expression as external to human language. Obviously when the human being hears the sheep bleat, language can be said to emerge and develop in a wholly human realm, namely, the soul into which the characteristic mark is sonically imprinted. The sheep's bleating, however, also serves to retain a central element from the language of sensations. Human language comes into being when the human being hears and responds to the primordial animal-human language. The clearly human act of reflection emerges subsequently at the moment the human being experiences (not contemplates or thinks about, but feels) something of its own, and not the merely animal, original language of sensations. To return to Oliver's claim: the relevance of the sheep (or any other animal for that matter) lies not in how it demonstrates that man learns to be human from the animal but rather, in its bleating sound, in confronting the human being with himself, with their original language which is inseparable from that of the animal. In other words, humans find themselves in language and reflection only insofar as they find themselves in relation to an immediate expression that they share with the animal. The animal here features specifically with reference to the sound it makes (and not, say, to its warming wool or nourishing milk). Sound for Herder is responsible for the connection between the two languages, a necessary connection since, as he specifically indicates, human language cannot arise directly from the primordial language of sensation; it cannot simply develop out of it. The sheep's bleating is precisely what Herder needs to give an account of the complexity of the relations between the two languages.

Rousseau on Language and Pain

In his description of man's encounter with the bleating sheep (as opposed to the instinctual, animal engagement with it), Herder argues that reflective human language does not originate in a spoken word nor as part of a confrontation with another human interlocutor, that is, it does not emerge in a communicative and social setting. The human being's first word, according to Herder, is called forth by his encounter with the sound of the bleating sheep, which in turn, institutes an internal linguistic space. The human *soul,* and not the human *mouth*, is indispensable for the emergence of language. This translates, however, not into a purely solipsistic image of language. Despite the fundamental absence of a fellow human interlocutor, Herder makes a point of positioning speaking man within a life sphere, a world. The sense of hearing signifies precisely that: man has to hear the sheep's bleating in order for an internal linguistic movement to be set off. He also has to identify the sheep *again* (the Ah!—Aha! movement) in order for a word to be seared into his soul, creating a characteristic sonic mark.

Notwithstanding the acoustic weight of this scene, another important element of Herder's thought emerges: although human language is not grounded in communication or reference, it has everything to do with the world of which humankind is part. Considering Herder's lengthy discussion of the life spheres and humans' weakness in comparison to animals, the first word, rather than being a representation of an object (say, the sheep), signals the constitution of a human relation to the world, a relation that emerges in the *Treatise* against the background of the animal's relation to its surrounding. As a result, the human is re-created as having-a-world rather than being deprived of it. The ability to hear the bleating and allow its sound to enter the soul and impress itself on it signals a redefinition of the human being's relationship with the world, with his life sphere. The original word, therefore, is not about the sheep as object; it neither describes it nor communicates something about it. For Herder, language marks the distinctive way in which humanity is positioned in relation to the world. In this sense, though it figures as an important example, the sheep's bleating also carries the risk of misunderstanding. The sheep is important only insofar as it sets into motion the human ability to orient oneself in the world, to get hold and arrest the overwhelming flood of sensations. Language, in other words, fundamentally does not concern "aboutness" (reference or communication), but rather, it constitutes a relationship.[54]

This account of language as constituting the possibility of relationality as such is not unique to Herder. It appears in a contemporaneous account of the question of the origin of language, written by Jean Jacques Rousseau, one of Herder's foremost rivals in the *Treatise*. Herder attacks Rousseau several times, criticizing his theory of the origin of language for turning "human beings into animals" (*Treatise* 77/*AS* 711). Herder is not only critical of Rousseau's positions; he is also sarcastic, sometimes even scornful, referring to his ideas as "deceptively dazzling" and "a bubble which he drives along before him for a time but which to his own surprise bursts on his way" (*Treatise* 86/*AS* 720). Elsewhere he despairs, asking rhetorically who can "endure" Rousseau's lengthy, unnecessary "sermons" (*Treatise* 142/*AS* 787).[55] Herder contends that Rousseau's definition of the "natural human being" (i.e., "his phantom" Herder writes), suffers from a crucial indeterminacy: "On the one hand, [he] fobs off with the ability for reason; on the other hand, [he] gets invested with perfectibility, and indeed with perfectibility as a distinctive character trait" (*Treatise* 94/*AS* 730). Instead of defining human uniqueness by way of its singular composition of thought and perception (like his own use of Besonnenheit), Rousseau simply adds reason to a natural creature, whose difference from the animal Herder therefore cannot grasp. Either this creature is an animal and can therefore not possess language, or it is human in the first place (and "necessarily already had a language of the soul!, already possessed the art of thinking which created the art of speaking" [*Treatise* 95/*AS* 731]), namely, not an animal miraculously transformed into a human being by way of adding the faculty of reason to its otherwise animal nature.[56]

Although his criticism is viable to an extent, it is clear that for the most part, Herder uses Rousseau as a straw man in the presentation of his own argument. As a consequence, he misses some crucial and fascinating similarities between Rousseau's arguments and his own. Herder's criticism is directed toward Rousseau's *Discourse on Inequality* (generally known as the *Second Discourse*) (1754),[57] a text with which he was well familiar and of which he was highly critical. In my following discussion, however, I refer to two other texts by Rousseau which I find illuminating in the context of Herder's *Treatise*. The first is *Emile, or on Education* (published in 1762, then banned and publicly burned);[58] the second is *The Essay on the Origin of Languages in Which Melody and Musical Imitation Are Treated*,[59] a text published only posthumously (1781), almost ten years after Herder's *Treatise*, and therefore not known to Herder at the time of its writing. Given the very specific context of my discussion here, I do not intend to offer a new interpretation of Rousseau's philosophy of language, nor do I deal with Herder polemically, defending Rousseau's position in view of Herder's criticism. This digression serves me, rather, to cast light on some points in Rousseau's argument which I find important and illuminating for my interpretation of Herder's *Treatise*.[60]

In one of Herder's critical comments, he explains the problematics inherent in Rousseau's treatment of man's relationship to the world and the description of his capacities: "Posit the human being as the being that he is, with that degree of sensuality and that organization, in the universe: from all sides, through all senses, this universe streams upon him in sensations. [Not] through human senses? [Not] in a human way? Does this thinking being [not], therefore, in comparison with the animals, get less flooded?" (*Treatise* 86/*AS* 721). Herder is looking for what he thinks of as the "human way" of encountering the world which he does not find in Rousseau. This is, however, a rather partial and crude engagement with Roussau that misses out on some of the complexities of the latter's claims. I would like to follow up on these and propose to take a look at another relevant text which Herder does not address, namely, Rousseau's *Emile*.

In *Emile*, Rousseau gives a fascinating complementary account of such a flood of sensations and describes language as emerging in consequence of human beings' "discomforts." This description appears in the first book of *Emile*, when Emile is still an infant, that is, he does not speak as yet. Rousseau writes that the child initially has only one language "because he has, so to speak, only one kind of discomfort" (*Emile* 65). For the child, prior to attaining language, all needs, wants, pains, and sorrows join into one overwhelming feeling Rousseau refers to in terms of "discomfort" or "only one sensation of pain" (*Emile* 65). The child is incapable of differentiating between being hungry or cold, tired, or stirred. Rousseau describes human wants and pains as the marks the world leaves on the child's experience, when the world strikes it, so to speak: so long as children "are awake, they are almost unable to remain in an indifferent state. They sleep or are affected" (*Emile* 64).[61] The infant feels only one thing: that something in what Rousseau calls "his mode of being" causes him suffering and needs change, needs intervention. Devoid of language, the child is completely exposed to the world, unable to hold back the strong flood of sensations the world unleashes on him.[62]

It is interesting to contemplate this description against the backdrop of the more prevalent Romantic view of childhood, which hinges on the child's innocent, primordial, and original experience of the world. In the adult view of the child's concentrated, pure gaze, it affords a glimpse into a prelinguistic, blissful mode of experiencing the world, an experience no longer possible for one who has lost this unique gaze once language was gained. Rousseau, in Emile, offers an entirely different account: instead of being calm and composed, the prelinguistic stage (common to infant and savage) is marked by violent outbursts of pain, fear, and suffering. With the child's entrance into language, these pains gradually lessen as they come to enter the linguistic space of expression.[63]

This is the background to Rousseau's argument: language emerges as a shield against the overwhelming flood of perception. Only when equipped with language, is the child able to position itself facing the world rather than being completely submerged by it. Without proper linguistic distance from the world there is, so to speak, no world at all, or at least—the world cannot become part of human experience. Rousseau's argument here is strikingly similar to Herder's description of the difference between humans and animals in the context of the latter's discussion of the "life spheres." For Herder too, language is born from a human weakness, not strength, and he too formulates human frailty in terms of humans' relationship to their surrounding world. Herder introduces Besonnenheit as the capacity that determines the uniquely human way of encountering the world, allowing man to appropriate it from the overwhelming flood. For Rousseau, the story unfolds somewhat differently: the infant lacks language and is therefore unable to keep the world at bay or experience it as differentiated. Language not only shields or protects us by means of providing a barrier to absorb the shock of the immediate encounter with reality, but it also has the power to soothe this encounter and alter the very experience it yields. With this claim, Rousseau raises an issue that is also formative for Herder's argument: for both authors, the frailty of the not-yet speaking infant is not social or communicative in nature. It involves, rather, an impaired ability to experience the world. The authors do not formulate the intersection between language and world as semiotic: that is, a relationship in which language describes, refers to, or signifies the world. Rather, for both thinkers, the relationship between language and world evinces a conundrum: their linguistic abilities protect humans from the forceful flood of an allegedly preexisting world, but at the same time humans can only *have* a world insofar as they have language.[64]

It is worthwhile to turn to Agamben's idea of "infancy" here. Although Agamben mentions the term in relation to neither Herder nor Rousseau, his understanding of the interrelations between infancy, language, and experience is important in the context of my discussion. Agamben poses the question of experience as a linguistic problem, arguing that the two—language and experience—cannot be separated. The possibility of human experience is essentially linked with the acquisition of language, since experience "cannot merely be something which chronologically precedes language and which, at a certain point, ceases to exist in order to spill into speech. It is not a paradise which, at a certain moment, we leave for ever in order to speak; rather, it coexists in its origins with language—indeed, is itself constituted through the appropriation of it by language in each instance to produce the individual as subject."[65] There is, in other words, no extra-linguistic paradise, no possibility to experience outside language, or in-fantly (Agamben here refers directly to the Latin *infantia* designating the inability to speak, a state of being without language).[66] Agamben uses Humboldt's theory of language, specifically the latter's claim that our naïve image of a language-less human being who gradually and naturally formed its own language is a fantasy. According to Humboldt, humanity can never be separated from language; it is, rather, "language whereby man is defined as man."[67] On this Agamben elaborates that since it is only through language that the individual is constituted, there is no form of anteriority to language.

Rousseau's interesting use of pain as exemplary for the "flood" demonstrates an emergent reciprocity at the convergence between pain and language: language is constituted and comes about by pain, but pain is also re-formed and transmuted by language. When the child learns to speak, it also learns to feel; what changes therefore, are its sensations themselves and not only their expressions. Once we have subjected the sensation of pain to its linguistic expression, we also experience it differently. In this sense, the utterance "I am in pain" does not represent the pain but actually changes the very way pain affects us, how it is felt in and on our bodies. What lies below the threshold of intense pain can apparently dissolve into the utterance of the word "pain," that is, the physical sensation is mollified as it dissolves into language. Such expression, according to Rousseau, would be a new, "appropriate," or proportionate understanding and articulation of the experience of pain. Where there is a cry or scream of pain, it would signal not merely the presence of pain but its intensity as well.[68]

Yet even for Rousseau, such a replacement has the structure of a residue: "As soon as Emile has once said, 'It hurts,' very intense pains indeed will be needed to force him to cry" (*Emile* 77). In moments of extreme pain, the now-speaking child is overwhelmed by an intensity of pain that cannot be "replaced" with speech. With this, Rousseau sets a clear threshold beyond which linguistic substitution no longer operates; the sensation of pain can be enclosed and encompassed within the word "pain" only up to a certain degree. In cases of intense pain, no words will suffice to express the sensation in such a way that the sensation is, literally, expressed. At such a level of pain, even those possessing language will burst into inarticulate cries. This demonstrates how, despite his account of the development and progression of language, Rousseau still retains language's essential connection to its point of origin. Even after Emile acquires the linguistic capabilities to express his pain in words, he does not lose his ability and need to immediately voice his pain in an inarticulate and passionate manner.

Rousseau points to what he understands as two forms of expression here—the cry and the word: "When children begin to speak, they cry less. This is a natural progress. One language is substituted for the other. As soon as they can say with words that they are in pain, why would they say it with cries, except when the pain is too intense for speech to express it?" (*Emile* 77). With this, Rousseau not only refers to the transition from a state of nature to a socially constructed form of expression: from the natural inarticulate cry to socially constituted speech; but also, and more important, he suggests there is an unequivocal difference between cry and word. Rousseau here does not merely wish to point at two different forms of language; he has a more decisive claim at stake—namely, that these two languages are mutually exclusive. Speech does not represent the cry or even the sensation of pain; instead, it *replaces* them.[69] Rousseau's argument can almost read as if the very utterance of the word "pain" itself were powerful enough to weaken and soothe the intensity of the actual physical pain. Emile learns that speaking of his pain (instead of wildly screaming it out) is an acceptable social behavior. And learning to speak is always coupled with entry not only into language but also into the linguistic community. Over and beyond this, Rousseau's argument also implies, taking a somewhat Wittgensteinian turn, that for Emile, rather than consciously suppressing or smothering his cry of pain in order to behave "socially," he finds that the advent of speech actually alters the experience of pain. Here the interesting implication is that the child's entry into language also marks a reentry into its own world. In contrast with his discussion of the origin of language in the *Discourse*, in *Emile* Rousseau proposes a view that is neither limited to the representational, referential, and communicative functions of language nor to humans' ability to imitate nature with language (precisely what Herder criticizes). *Emile* offers a different argument: by acquiring language, the child acquires the world anew, becoming re-oriented and re-positioned within it; and more explicitly, the child now has a different *relation* to it.

This, I believe, is a key element in the present imagined encounter (or, re-encounter) between Herder and Rousseau. Language enables human beings to make distinctions in a world that assails their exposed senses.[70] Similar to Herder's uniquely human Besonnenheit, which differentiates a wave, singling it out as something with which the soul entertains a relationship, Rousseau's formulation of language provides us with an account in which the child's acquisition of language marks his having a world and, simultaneously, being able to orient himself within it. One intriguing aspect of this understanding of language is that here language appears not only as a relationship but also as providing the human being with a type of *measure* or yardstick. Rousseau invokes this idea in a long and telling footnote in the second book of *Emile*, where he cites Buffon's *Histoire Naturelle* to elucidate some points in his own discussion of fear and specifically his claim that fear is a consequence of "ignorance of the things which surround us and of what is going on about us" (*Emile* 134). Buffon's writings offer an interesting account of how the initial appearance of objects around us may be far more threatening and frightful than they "really" are, as Rousseau formulates it. Using examples such as horses, flies, and sheep (!), Buffon explains how our misjudging of the proper distance between us and the object of experience can directly affect our perception, or more precisely, determine whether our perception is "appropriate." Rousseau quotes Buffon as follows: "From this come the terror and kind of inner fear that the darkness of night causes almost all men to feel. On this is founded the appearance of specters and gigantic, frightful figures that so many people say they have seen. . . . This must, indeed, surprise and frighten him up until he finally gets to touch the object or to recognize it, for at the very instant he recognizes what it is, the object which appeared gigantic will suddenly diminish and will no longer appear to be anything but its real size" (*Emile* 134–135 fn.).

Although language is not at the center of Buffon's discussion, his argument is nevertheless thought provoking in regard to Rousseau's account of pain and fear. What Buffon describes as "mastery" of the experience of the world by the "correction" or counterbalance one must make of one's initial, inaccurate, and inappropriate experience is precisely echoed in Rousseau's discussion of the relationship between the sensation of pain and its articulation in words. In Buffon's account, fear of an unknown gigantic object in the dark provides us, first, with an "inappropriate" perception and judgment; only subsequently, this inappropriate perception may transform into knowledge of the object's appropriate or proper nature, so that it can be recognized for "what it is" (not a monster but a sheep). In Rousseau's account, however, unlike in Buffon's, the correction or transformation of the initial overwhelming sensation into a manageable and confined linguistic utterance is achieved not by observation but as a result of the very acquisition of language. Buffon's notion of the inappropriateness of our perceptions in the dark reappears in Rousseau's account, referring this time not to the dark of night but to the dark of language-less-ness. For Rousseau, the correction of experience, the moment in which we can make the experience "appropriate" or neutralize it, is a *purely linguistic moment.* Our perception of the world as well as our experience of pain or fear, in this example, can only become *appropriate* when they are *appropriated* by language.

Language as Relation: Herder and Rousseau

This notion of language as first replacing the initial feeling or emotive reaction, and second, being capable of assuaging or "down-sizing" the intensity of the reaction, can also be found in Rousseau's *Essay on the Origin of Languages.* In the celebrated third chapter of the *Essay* ("That the first language must have been figurative"), Rousseau is preoccupied with figurative and literal language, tackling the question of precedence, or in this case, which came first. Rousseau argues that figurative language precedes literal language, and, moreover, that literal language can only appear after the figurative, emotive encounter with the world has initiated the first linguistic utterance (*Essay* 253–254). But here, Rousseau encounters a logical difficulty: how can figurative expression, usually considered to be constructed around literal meaning, in fact precede an object's literal meaning (which Rousseau also calls "proper meaning")? How can the metaphoric and figurative expression be a *condition* for a "proper" or "true" linguistic utterance, rather than the other way around? To account for this problem and justify his argument, Rousseau provides an example:

> A savage meeting others will at first have been frightened. His fright will have made him see these men as larger and stronger than himself; he will have called them *Giants.* After much experience he will have recognized that since these supposed Giants are neither bigger nor stronger than he, their stature did not fit the idea that he had initially attached to the word Giant. He will therefore invent another name common both to them and to himself, for example the name *man,* and he will restrict the name *Giant* to the false object that had struck him during his illusion. This is how the figurative word arises before the proper [or literal] word does, when passion holds our eyes spellbound and the first idea which it presents to us is not that of the truth. (*Essay* 254)

I suggest that we read this passage in light of Rousseau's argument in *Emile*. What we have here is not a child but a savage, whose role in the story is that of a "child of humanity," or one in his pre-social, infantile phase (literally "infantile": the inability to use language). Here Rousseau describes the savage's very first encounter with another human being. This is a surprising and passionate moment giving rise to a strong emotional response that takes the form of fear.[71] The intensity of this fear leads the savage to construe the other as "larger and stronger" than himself. The resulting utterance marks a moment in which, in Rousseau's words, "passion holds our eyes spellbound," or in a different translation, "our gaze is held in passionate fascination" (*Essay* 254). This fascination does not lead to language but rather to a play of images that keeps language suspended. Language can only begin when this spell of fascination is broken. "Giant" is hence neither a linguistic description nor some other representation of the object encountered. It is an expression that completely escapes any propositional or communicative structure, giving voice to the deep fear the encounter with the other arouses.[72]

The first utterance, "giant," according to Rousseau, fails in two significant ways: first, it fails to *differentiate* the encountered object (a man) from the overwhelming passion it induced (fear); and second, it fails in accurately judging the nature, and especially the size, of the object at hand. Rephrased in terms of Rousseau's initial problem, when the savage first encounters another man, his initial word "giant" expresses figurative meaning, whereas the following word "man" indicates the literal or "proper" meaning of the object. The essential error or misjudgment is expressed in the word "giant," which is later *corrected* in the word "man." Rousseau sums up his example as follows: "Since the illusory image presented by passion showed itself first, the language answering to it was invented first; subsequently it became metaphorical when the enlightened mind recognized its original error and came to use expressions of that first language only when moved by the same passion as had produced it" (*Essay* 254). But this important example not only establishes Rousseau's argument regarding the relationship between figurative and literal meaning. I want to suggest here that it also, and foremost, demonstrates something about the structure of language itself. The word "giant" did not, in effect, refer to the other man at all; rather, the word referred to the *passion* that the encounter with the other man induced, namely, fear. Only when the feeling itself has subsided, when it is "purged" of the distortion of the initial emotive response, can the described object receive its "proper" or "true" name: "man."

This might clarify Rousseau's insistence on the primacy of the figurative. If the figurative or metaphorical is the way in which language expresses something by means of its relation to something else— and marks language's return to the object *through* something else—then, the possibility of saying "man" can only become feasible after "giant" is expressed. It is in this sense, as Friedlander points out in his discussion of Rousseau's *Reveries of a Solitary Walker*, the vehemence of the strong passions might suggest an excess of meaning, inherent to language itself: "To face the predicament, to be truthful in the face of such excess, would demand in the first place letting yourself be exposed to it. . . . [T]he exposure to meaning requires precisely giving up intention, withstanding the excess."[73] A proportionate linguistic appraisal of the object at hand can therefore only come about with the counterbalancing or evening-out of the excessive expression of passion. Friedlander continues to explain that the linguistic detour by which the figurative has the power to return us to its object by way of something else, ostensibly false, is in fact necessary when there is no way to speak directly of the thing itself.[74]

Comparing this argumentation with the former discussion of pain in *Emile*, we can trace a configuration in which Rousseau's *psychological* intuitions about the child prior to his entry into language (in *Emile*) are adapted into *linguistic* ones (in the *Essay*). The replacement of the child's inarticulate cry with a word is consummately echoed by the substitution of "giant" with "man." In both cases, the substitution essentially has a soothing or calming effect, with the initial excess of feeling neutralized through the equanimity or composure of the word. The first cry or exclamation of fear—here the word "giant" is considered an exclamation, not a word—marks a heightened emotional response. The second utterance, however—whether a sentence "I'm in pain" or the new word "man"—is a composed, "collected" utterance, expressing the neutralization of the initial strong emotive response.

But Rousseau's explanation of the way in which the linguistic utterance "downsizes" the object, restoring it to its "true size"— takes into account only the measures of the object at stake (the other human being or, in *Emile*, the child's specific want). The linguistic sign representing this object indeed transforms from the figurative to the literal, and thus, precisely confirms Rousseau's hypothesis about the primacy of the figurative. But what this account overlooks is that the initial utterance can be considered unfit only insofar as the *object* at hand is concerned, but *not* when it refers to the emotion that this object induces in the subject. That is to say, when the child cries or the savage exclaims "giant," these expressions might be linguistic exaggerations in reference to the object of expression (whether hunger or man), but they are a perfectly accurate rendering of the child's or savage's emotive and passionate response to it. The hungry or tired child *in fact* cries out in pain, and the savage is *undeniably* scared. Articulate language can be said to enter the passionate scene so as to downsize the appearance of the object or neutralize the terror with which it strikes us; what it describes, however, is not the object itself (that can now be "resized") but rather the passion (in our case, fear, pain, or a more general experience of suffering). "Giant," therefore, denotes fear whereas "man" points at another human being, similar in size, confronting the savage. The transformation of the child's cry and the savage's exclamation into "literal" or "true sized" words is therefore not merely a transition between different languages as Rousseau has it; it relates, rather, to a change in language's very object of reference: instead of referring to the object encountered, it refers to the passion engendered in the speaker by the encounter.

In his famous interpretation of this scene,[75] Derrida explains the importance of the "inadequacy" of metaphor:

> it is the *inadequation of the designation* (metaphor) which *properly expresses* the passion. If fear makes me see giants where there are only men, the signifier—as the idea of the object—will be metaphoric, but the signifier of my passion will be literal. And if I then say "I see giants," that false designation will be a literal expression of my fear. For in fact I see giants and there is a sure truth there."[76]

Derrida's emphasis here is on the unique way in which the true (affect) comes together with the false (reference to an object), forming the metaphoric structure: the word "giant" might be a false or inadequate designation of the object (another man) yet it is a proper and thereby literal expression of the passion that this object induces in the savage (fear). The word "giant" refers, therefore, not to the object standing before the savage but rather the fearsome manner in which the other man appeared before the savage, namely, *as* giant, fearsome, stronger, and so on.

This is the meaning of Derrida's aforementioned claim about the inadequation of the designation: fear is, therefore, not an object in itself, nor does it arise from the mere difference in size between the two men. It is the inadequacy itself that expresses the fear, so that the gap between (1) the signifier's inadequacy in relation to the signified, and (2) its adequacy and accuracy in regard to what the object in fact induces in me (fear)—this very gap represents the structure of passion. Derrida criticizes positions that situate the passions somehow within the subject, as if it were some internal "content" that is then, in turn, expressed linguistically: "The fact that 'giant' is literal as sign of fear not only does not prevent, but on the contrary implies, that it should be nonliteral or metaphoric as sign of the object. It cannot be the idea-sign of the passion without presenting itself as the idea-sign of the presumed cause of that passion, opening an exchange with the outside."[77] Fear is not *in* the subject and not *in* the object: it emerges from the gap between them or perhaps inheres in the moment the speaking subject experiences the object. Derrida's claim implies that language does not represent the passion qua object, since the passion is always about a relationship between people, man, and world, and so forth. The vehemence of passion is felt, and represented, only from within a difference, a gap. Derrida's account is not only consequential for our understanding of Rousseau but also pertinent in that it provides a perspective on the nature of the encounter between passions and language in general: passions emerge from, and appear in, the in-between, in the relation, and therefore cannot be captured or expressed with a demonstrative gesture, as referential content.

In his critique of Derrida,[78] Paul de Man accuses him of producing an interpretation that dangerously resembles Rousseau's own text. However, instead of reading the "real" Rousseau, he deconstructs a "pseudo-Rousseau," thus providing what de Man calls "a classical case of critical blindness."[79] De Man agrees with Derrida that the word "giant" "may be objectively false (the other man is not in fact any taller) but it is subjectively candid (he seems taller to the frightened subject); the statement may be an error but it is not a lie, as it "expresses" the inner experience correctly."[80] However, de Man criticizes Derrida for remaining trapped in the traditional understanding of passion as a kind of bridging between inside and outside when he claims that "giant" refers to an inner feeling of fear. According to de Man, Derrida fails to understand that the reason for fear has to do with a concrete appearance of something in the external world, with "observable data" (de Man understands Derrida as offering an internal state of affairs as fear's object, a disputable interpretation). Fear results from a fundamental distrust: what appears before me is a man who seems similar to me in size, yet despite this apparent similarity, he may in fact pose a threat. In other words, fear is the result of my suspecting a *possible* discrepancy between the external and internal properties of entities and has to do with an inherent "fear" that things are not as they appear to be, that the "reassuringly familiar and similar outside might be a trap."[81]

De Man offers an alternative understanding of the function of passions and emotions by employing an epistemic frame of reference:

> The fear of another man is hypothetical; no one can trust a precipice, but it remains an open question, for whoever is neither a paranoiac nor a fool, whether one can trust one's fellow man. By calling him a "giant" one freezes hypothesis, or fiction, into fact and makes fear, itself a figural state of suspended meaning, into a definite, proper meaning devoid of alternatives. The metaphor "giant," used to connote man, has indeed a proper meaning (fear), but this meaning is not really proper: it refers to a condition of permanent suspense between a literal world in which appearance and nature coincide and a figural world in which this correspondence is no longer a priori posited. Metaphor is error because it believes or feigns to believe in its own referential meaning.[82]

For de Man, "giant" refers to a moment of epistemic suspension or indeterminacy. It therefore designates neither the object nor the passion but the epistemic oscillation between the two. The savage uses the word "giant" to refer to the man facing him, but what the word actually designates is the state of a suspension of meaning within which the savage finds himself, overwhelmed by fear.

De Man criticizes Derrida for using passion to compensate for the inherent discrepancy between the outward appearances of objects and their "true" inner properties, since for de Man, this discrepancy is precisely what cannot be resolved. For Rousseau, de Man continues, "all passions—whether they be love, pity, anger, or even a borderline case between passion and need such as fear—are characterized by such a discrepancy; they are based not on the knowledge that such a difference exists, but on the hypothesis that it might exist, a possibility that can never be proven or disproven by empirical or by analytical means. A statement of distrust is neither true nor false: it is rather in the nature of a permanent hypothesis."[83] De Man's argument in these last lines illuminates something crucial about the relationship between language and the passions: our fear or distrust does not stem from an actual breach or contradiction. It originates, rather, from the *possibility* that such a discrepancy exists. "Giant" therefore, does not designate an object or its size, or even what I feel toward it; it expresses, rather, the potential risk that what I see is not, so to speak, what I get. This potential is clearly inherent in, and essential to, language as such. The origin of language cannot be discussed without taking into account this risk.[84]

It is no wonder then, that Rousseau chose to focus on problems of proportion (whether problems of a disproportionate evaluation of size or an allegedly exaggerated emotive response). Such problems highlight the fact that language is always about an encounter with an *other* (whether man, animal, or object) and is therefore always an expression of a relationship between speaking man and something or someone other than himself, a way to assess and express the implications of such an encounter. (This is also true where languages do not communicate outwardly but express "inner content" such as feelings and thought; this would be what Herder refers to as cases of the "soul speaking to itself"). Moreover, as Bruns attentively remarks, fear and pain are the "hidden meaning of all human speech, as if it were so that the very words I am speaking now contained a secret expression of fear."[85] Fear and pain are therefore the latent but fundamental content of human speech, its point of origin but also, and foremost, its innermost nature. Rather than ignoring it as merely nostalgic, Rousseau retains the emotional, original linguistic utterance as the infra-structure of language as such—a structure that is revealed in extreme moments of passion and linguistic moments alike: in the experience of deep suffering, in intense pain, as well as (and not less important!) in figurative and metaphoric language. What all these moments share is that they touch on an extreme; pushing the limits of the human ability to bear its suffering and to give it expression. In this sense my reading of Rousseau crucially figures moments in which language itself, and not only the feeling of suffering, reaches its limits. In these moments, where language does not function as a mere signifying apparatus, something essential about its origin and internal structure stands revealed. And the same goes for the very experience of being human: its contours grow sharp and its nature unfolds only at its extremes, when it strikes the limits of the experience of being human—and suffering is one such salient limit.

My point in bringing together Rousseau and Herder is that the word "giant," much like the sheep's bleating, demonstrates that in language the object and its impression cannot, essentially, be experienced in isolation from one another. Therein lies the uniqueness of Herder's and Rousseau's theories of language. For both, language constructs a space of experience whose configuration does not enable crude distinctions between objects, perceptions, and affects. Rousseau's savage fearing the giant other, as well as Herder's bleating which is forcefully imprinted on the human soul, demonstrate precisely this. The bleating sheep is perhaps singled out and separated from the flood of sensations by the human being who has language, but it is not and cannot be separated from this same human being who experiences it. The word "giant" expresses neither the other man as object nor the passion that it induces in the speaker; it is a vehement exclamation expressing the passionate content of the *encounter itself*—savage and other man, man and bleating sheep—experienced in an indivisible linguistic expanse. Moreover, both thinkers similarly contemplate the problematic inherent in the encounter between language and passion. Considering such an encounter in terms of the relationship between language and pain, we could say that for both Herder and Rousseau, the question at hand is not so much whether language is capable or incapable of fully or accurately encapsulating a given sensation or passion. Rather, for both Herder and Rousseau, the strong eruption of passion becomes the condition of possibility for the emergence of linguistic expression. This is not because language is capable of representing or referring to the passion but because the latter provides an extreme case in the face of which alone language can emerge.

4

Language and Hearing

Heidegger's Herder

Heidegger's Herder

Pain evolves and issues forth from a unique internal incongruity that can be described in terms of movement: on the one hand, the experience of pain is accompanied by a movement outward and away from the suffering body and into the realm shared by others. This reaching out is markedly sonic in nature, as the agonized body cries out its pain, as if trying to discard its physical agony by expressing it in distraught cries that reach every ear, no matter how distant. Rather than being dependent on a preexisting responsive community, this outward-bound movement of pain's expression, can be said to constitutes a community. The experience of pain coincides therefore with transcendence from the private, solipsistic self. On the other hand, pain is distinguished by an opposite movement. It violently drives us inward, enclosing us within our suffering body with no way out, mesmerizing us by its intensity. No one is allowed entrance; no one understands or can genuinely *know* our pain. It cannot be shared or distributed. It is our very own; it becomes us.

The pained human body, wedged between these two antithetical movements, is dismembered and at the same time inevitably shared in expression. This singular configuration of pain is not to be understood merely as a collision between the individual and his or her pain, between volition and instinct, human and animal. Pain is distinguished precisely by its paradoxical nature, by the fact that any thinking that surrenders to mutually exclusive structures lacks the power to grasp pain's singular nature.

This conundrum of pain is borne out in the relationship between the *Treatise*'s first two sections, or between Herder's two languages: the primary language of sensations, which is animal-human, and reflective, human language. The first is immediate, instinctive, and markedly sonic in nature; its crux is the human and animal voice calling out its pain in expressive cries and screams. The paragraphs in which Herder speaks of the sympathy of nature (*Treatise* 66/*AS* 698) can be understood to instigate a shared, communal space in which cries of pain and an overwhelming, immediate sympathy come together at one stroke. Even when the presence of a sympathetic interlocutor is in doubt or denied, the suffering animal or human (or, for that matter, Philoctetes) cries out. In the case of the language of sensations, therefore, the experience of pain is conceived of and described in terms of its expression, actualized outside the confines of the suffering body (human or animal), rather than existing as an "internal" content. This expressive language of sensations transforms in the second section of the *Treatise* into distinctly human, reflective, and markedly *non-sonic* language. Human language and Besonnenheit do not appear in the second part of Herder's *Treatise* related to the production of voice or any other form of sonic expression: quite the contrary, human language emerges as a human attitude toward the world, a relationship between humans and their life circle, and finally, a silent movement between humans and themselves, or in Herder's words, a state in which the "soul speaks to itself."

Herder's two languages seem to proffer a structure that consists of opposing movements: an outward, immediate, and strong sound-bearing movement of expression, and an inner, *silent* movement of the soul withdrawing so as to encounter itself and thereby creating an inner word. A close look reveals that these oppositions in fact operate on a similar pitch. The structure of sympathy and response occurring in the external realm, outside the pained body, is met with a parallel structure of resonance and response that occurs within. As we have already seen, this division between the two languages is not a simply binary as Herder seems to present it, and moreover, his attempts to move between the two linguistic formations are not sufficiently grounded and justified. Suspended between the first two sections of the *Treatise,* Herder seems to be wrestling with a quandary: he declares a breach between the two languages, however, he concurrently portrays them as exceedingly correspondent.

One may approach this problematic from a critical perspective, to reveal a weakness in Herder's argument, then to call for alternatives either substantiating the division of the *Treatise* into two sections or rendering them compatible. My approach to this manifest split in Herder's *Treatise* is different. I suggest we consider it not in terms of a weakness or mistake on Herder's part, trying to "save" Herder from his own error, but rather, to think of his theory from a broader perspective that holds together the diversity as well as interconnection between the two sections. The problem of the relationship between the two languages reflects a breach inherent in the experience of pain as such. It is in this sense that I take the *Treatise* to be paradigmatic for my own thinking about pain and its relationship to language: it opens an important view not only on the experience of pain and its expression but also, and more important, on its internal paradoxes, breaches, and rifts. Just as pain is both expressive and solipsistic, both sonic and silently enclosed, so too, is the configuration of Herder's two languages.

The problem of the relationship between Herder's two languages forms the core of "On the Essence of Language: The Metaphysics of Language and the Essencing of the Word" (*Vom Wesen der Sprache: Die Metaphysik der Sprache und die Wesung des Wortes*),[1] a seminar that Martin Heidegger taught at the University of Freiburg in the winter of 1939.[2] Other than a short introduction to the traditional problem of the origin of language and some discussions of G. W. Leibniz, Jacob Grimm, and Stefan George (representing philosophical, philological, and poetic points of view, respectively), the greater part of the seminar is devoted to a close reading of Herder's *Treatise* (the seminar's subtitle is "Concerning Herder's Treatise on the Origin of Language"). One of Heidegger's main objectives in the *Seminar* is to distinguish between Herder's question of the *origin* of language (which he takes to be a metaphysical question) and that of the *essence* of language (a question that, according to Heidegger, overcomes metaphysics in favor of the question of being). "Is language and its essence explained and graspable through the meditation on the origin?" Heidegger asks, "Does the proof of the origin ever guarantee the knowledge of the essence"? (*Seminar-N* 72/*WS* 84). Heidegger's worry is that the very posing of the question as one of origin will essentially "lock" the possibility to inquire into (and experience) the essence of language (*Seminar-N* 73/*WS* 85)—language should be approached from the perspective of being, not mere genealogy. Heidegger claims that Herder's approach to origin is metaphysical insofar as his project involves a transcendence of language in search of an external "anchor" from which its beginning can be determined. Heidegger elaborates on this in *Contributions of Philosophy*, in which he explicitly argues that the search for "the" a-historical language, diffuses the question of essence, which "immediately appear[s] to swirl confusedly."[3] Posing the question of origin, he continues, cannot lead us beyond the metaphysical sphere of language as an external, instrumental apparatus that is merely *related* or belongs to man, rather than being his very essence. Heidegger differentiates between the metaphysical-anthropological conception of language (language as assertion, representation, and tool) and his own approach, according to which the overcoming of metaphysics has the power to free the question of the truth of being from any explanations that resort to transcendence or an "ideal" language (*Contributions* 353–354 [501–502]).

Heidegger's alternative, when he suggests to overcome metaphysics, seeks to ground the essence of language from within itself. Such a procedure would determine first, language itself, and only then its metaphysical explanation (*Contributions* 351 [498]). The *Seminar* demonstrates a similar course of argument: the problem lies in Herder's very *search* for origins, not in his findings. Although his path runs very close to the question of essence, Herder poses the question in a way that limits the possible scope of his answer. Heidegger explains this in the *Seminar* as follows: "The metaphysical question of essence [Wesensfrage] is always [a] question of origin [Herkunftsfrage]. . . . The origin is not yet found, but only the place of what has sprung [Entsprungenen], something 'that has sprung' *found*, where something of the essence of language [is made] visible" [sichtbar] (*Seminar-N* 83, 127/*WS* 97, 148). These observations serve Heidegger to establish his entry point into his interpretation of Herder, which will take different paths throughout the *Seminar*. But before I delve into the details of Heidegger's criticism of Herder, a few words about the text of the *Seminar* are required.

The published version of the *Seminar* can by no means be treated as an organized, complete philosophical interpretation of Herder. We only have Heidegger's preparatory notes (sometimes presented as numbered lists or extremely condensed outlines, at other times in diagrams) and class transcripts taken by eleven students who attended the seminar. While it is at times possible to trace the connection between Heidegger's own preparatory notes and the transcripts, this connection is usually very loose (not to mention the fact that each student took down notes of a different class). In the retrospections he write after the seminar, Heidegger refers to these class transcripts remarking that

> the actual course of the classes cannot always be gleaned from them; this insight is provided by the "Notes," each of which always has a different "value," and even there where they report "literally" never present the questions just as I had completely characterized and talked them over.[4]

This has a twofold implication: the transcripts are not always in line with Heidegger's preliminary notes, yet it is precisely because of this that they provide us with a useful elaboration on these, sometimes extremely vague, notes.[5] This said, the *Seminar* is nevertheless an indispensable source, not only for our understanding of Heidegger's later philosophy and Herder's strong influence on him but also since it sheds an interesting light on some of the central problems in Herder's *Treatise*. Heidegger makes a point of demonstrating, again and again and from different angles and discursive perspectives, that the *Treatise* is not strong enough philosophically, that it falls prey to a long Western philosophical tradition that approaches language from a metaphysical outlook. This is a view on language as instrument, a communicative, representational apparatus yielding claims only *about* the world or in reference to it.

But despite his fierce, sometimes confrontational, criticism of Herder, one cannot escape feeling that Heidegger is exceedingly interested in the *Treatise*. He is clearly attracted to Herder's line of argument, his examples, and even his errors, into which he delves in great detail, critically yet lovingly. Heidegger's interest in Herder is, however, not only expressed in the *Seminar*: a close look at Heidegger's work reveals references to Herder in several places, and although they are usually minor and made in passing, they mark Herder's presence throughout his work, from *What Are Poets For?* (1926), *Being and Time* (1927) and *The Fundamental Concepts of Metaphysics* (1929–1930). The *Seminar* stands out in this respect. It is the only text in which Heidegger rigorously, even if critically, focuses on Herder's thought. As some interpreters such as Taylor or Kovacs have argued, there is no doubt that Herder had a strong, profound influence on Heidegger's ideas. Referring to this influence, Sikka claims that it is characteristic for Heidegger to not fully acknowledge his debt to other philosophers (Aristotle and Hegel are prominent examples).[6]

The Problem

There are different ways into the maze of the *Seminar*. For one thing, there is Heidegger's explicit criticism of Herder's "metaphysical" outlook on language and the allegedly narrow angle from which the latter views the origin and essence of human language. Another start would be Heidegger's repeated attempts to undermine what he takes to be Herder's understanding of human language as originating from his conception of man as *animal rationale*, an animal to which language is added, like some external adornment. There is also the encounter Heidegger stages between Herder's theory of language and Grimm or Humboldt, or the peculiar section about Stefan George's poetry. My approach to the text, however, takes the vantage point of *sound*. Heidegger is an avid and rigorous reader of Herder throughout the text, but it is in his analysis of what he calls "the sound character of language," that his contribution to our understanding of Herder's conception of language is most rewarding. Sound for Heidegger is central in two ways: first, he identifies the main problematics in the *Treatise* in terms of sound, pointing at an incongruity between Herder's different definitions of language as being acoustic and nonacoustic at the same time; second, he formulates his own response by means of an elaborate network of terms closely associated with sound and hearing. Let me start with Heidegger's formulation of the problem.[7]

The first difficulty Heidegger identifies in the *Treatise* is an inconsistency between its notions of a primary human-animal language of sensations and a distinctly human language of reflective awareness. Herder begins the first section of the *Treatise* with the words, "Already as an animal the human being has language" (*Treatise* 65/*AS* 697), whereas in the second section he writes that "human beings are the only linguistic creatures that we know, and are distinguished from all the animals precisely by language" (*Treatise* 77/*AS* 711). Heidegger comments that, on the one hand, Herder presents the human being as an animal possessing a nonverbal language, made up of cries, sighs, and screams of pain. On the other hand, the human is *distinguished* from the animal by having a language, that is, a nonanimal language, developed later in the text as inherently connected, if not identical, with human reflective abilities (Besonnenheit), thereby construing language as an apparatus that operates in the human soul. To put this in terms of sound, language is characterized by way of two conflicting definitions: a language of *sound* composed of instinctive cries and immediate expressions of pain; and a decidedly *silent* language, distinctly human in being an attitude and relationship toward the world and human life circles that relies on the inner movement of the human soul in its formation of a characteristic mark (*Merkmal*) and inner word (*Innere Wort*) (*Seminar-N* 3–4/*WS* 3–4; *Seminar-T* 134, 136/*WS* 157–158, 158–159).

The second important difficulty in the *Treatise*'s line of argument as pointed out by Heidegger again involves the problematics of sound. The human being, perceiving and listening to the sound of the bleating sheep, is able to distinguish it from the object that produces the sound (the sheep) and, eventually, to turn it into the first word of his language. The sound dimension inherent in the origin of human language dominates Herder's description of the scene. By introducing human reflective awareness or Besonnenheit, however, Herder departs from the sensory dimension of sound and turns to what he describes as the "inner word of the soul." This is when the sheep's bleating transforms into an internal bleating that "rings out" (*es klang*) in a "resounding word" (*tönendes Wort*) (*Treatise* 98/*AS* 734). This development is central to Herder's claim since according to the *Treatise,* "even if the human being's tongue had never tried to stammer it . . . still his soul has, so to speak, bleated internally" [in ihrem Inwendigen geblöckt] (*Treatise* 89/*AS* 724). This transformation, or even conversion, of the *sonorous* (sheep's bleating) into the *nonsonorous* (Besonnenheit and the internal bleating of the soul) reappears when Herder needs to explain the possibility of a progression or translation from the inner word and characteristic mark into the spoken word, discourse, and communication.

These two ambiguities instigate Heidegger's forthright attack on Herder:

> [Herder] does not succeed in grasping the essence of the human being as reflective awareness in a unified and general manner; he does not succeed in leaving the traditional determination of the human being as animal rationale. . . . And as Herder does not succeed, even if he also aims at this, in grasping the human being in his essence (thinking and sensibility) in a uniform manner and thus in contrasting him essentially against the animal, he does not succeed in deriving the word in its

double structure in a uniform manner. Thus, verbal language remains only a certain kind of sonorous, communicating expression in contrast with the animal's voice, the cry of sensation, and is not essentially distinguished from it, although the claim for such an essential distinction is made. And if *Herder* says . . . that in order to explain the origin of language it is decisive to know what reason is, then one can say that Herder did not know what reason really is. (*Seminar-T* 166–167/*WS* 203–204)

According to Heidegger, Herder's twofold determination of human language (or "word," as he refers to it here) as sonorous expression, on the one hand, and inner nonsonorous, on the other, fails to provide a unified account of the human being (he uses the phrase "does not succeed" four times in this passage alone). In consequence, Herder's explicit claim for the essential distinction between man and animal remains thoroughly unestablished and, more important, portrays animal and human language as differing merely in degree rather than in kind. This failure—in Heidegger's reading—firmly places Herder within the Western philosophical tradition in which the human being is conceived as an animal to which reason, and thereby language, is added: an *animal rationale.* Heidegger's criticism of this idea appears already in *Being and Time* (1927) where he writes that the definition of the human as an *animal rationale* is perhaps not entirely false but only partially touches on the definition of *Dasein*: "The human being shows himself as a being who speaks. This does not mean that the possibility of vocal utterance belongs to him, but that this being is in the mode of discovering world and Da-sein itself" (*BT* 155 [165]).[8] In an attempt to follow similar lines and challenge what he takes to be Herder's limited definition of language, Heidegger suggests here that we don't take Herder's divisions and conceptual distinctions at face value and attempt instead to read between them or, rather, transcend them so as to recover a more unified, stable conception of language as well as of man. As Heidegger phrases it in one of his notes: "Not divine, not animalistic, but 'human'!! That says only: language characterizes the human being—but who is the human being?" [Sprache zeichnet den Menschen aus—aber wer ist der Mensch?] (*Seminar-N* 39/*WS* 48).[9] Heidegger tackles this problem by arguing that the unity lacking between both Herder's two languages as well as the two split parts of the human being, can only be found when considering "the whole of the treatise" in a single stroke (*Seminar-T* 136/*WS* 160).

Let us, then, tie the threads of the argument together. Heidegger identifies two central problems in the *Treatise*: first, Herder presents two categorically different creatures—animal and man—but his account of the exact difference or even the mere relationship between them remains inconsistent; second, Herder describes two types of language: an outreaching, sound-bearing form of linguistic expression (cry, scream, word) and an internal, silent language of *Merkmal,* attention, and reflection. Heidegger shows that in neither case Herder provides sufficient ground to account for the transition between the two—animal and human, inner and outer, sonorous and nonsonorous language—and he claims that Herder is unable to provide a coherent conceptualization of the speaking human being. But it is not a mere critical analysis of Herder's *Treatise* that Heidegger is looking for. The *Seminar* sets out to use these inherent problems in Herder's theory as a steppingstone for Heidegger's own alternative conception of language. While Heidegger stays very close to the *Treatise*'s formulations and concepts, he takes us a long way from Herder's original claims.

The "Sound Character" of Language

Having broached the possibility to account for the *Treatise* as a whole, Heidegger poses a crucial question: "how can the nonsonorous marks become sound?" (*Seminar-T* 160/*WS* 195), or in other words, how is the sheep's bleating sound transformed into an inner word of the soul, and thence, how can this inner word become, eventually, sonorous speech? What is the relationship between the *linguistic* silent inner movement of the soul and the audible linguistic apparatus that we usually think of when we think about language? The solution to these problems lies, according to Heidegger, in the sound character of language (*Lautcharakter der Sprache*), a solution foregrounded by Herder himself, albeit without its being his explicit intention, and without being a "completely secured" solution (*Seminar-T* 155/*WS* 187). Herder goes only halfway; as a result, "the problem of [the] sound character of language is not solved, the connection between inner and outer word is not grasped in its ground" (*Seminar-T* 166/*WS* 204). Since Herder "merely" foregrounds sound but fails to develop and establish his argument, Heidegger takes up this task in the *Seminar*. The sound character of language is central to Heidegger's argument, since it is here that the conflicting ends of Herder's argument—inner as well as outer, sonorous and nonsonorous—can be brought together. It is precisely the sound character of language that "makes possible the necessary *crossing-over* from inner to outer word," "the silent inner resounding word as well as the elements of spoken language" (*Seminar-T* 155/*WS* 187, my emphasis, trans. modified). Heidegger introduces a crucial term here: *Übergang*.

Before I continue, a short note on translation is in place. The standard English translation of Übergang is "transition" (such a translation appears, for instance, in Heidegger's *Contributions to Philosophy (of the Event)* and his Nietzsche lectures of the same period).[10] However, Wanda Torres, and Gregory and Yvonne Unna, the translators of the *Seminar*, use "crossing" instead. This is, I assume, first and foremost because of Heidegger's own argument as for the necessity to abandon what he calls the traditional understanding of Übergang as "the transitory." Heidegger wants to emphasize the *experience* of the Übergang itself rather than the change or transformation it brings about. "Crossing," however, neglects the element of *Über*, the over, of the crossing. This is important insofar as the two ends crossed, the in-between, should be retained, and should remain part of the experience of the crossing itself.[11] In order to be faithful to what I take to be Heidegger's intention in Übergang, I will hereafter use "crossing-over."

The crossing-over in Heidegger's argument constitutes an intermediate space: not entirely sonorous, it is also not nonsonorous; neither utterly silent nor yet merely expressive. He gives an interesting (yet vague and complicated) account of the term in the *Seminar*, criticizing the approach that treats the crossing-over as a transitory space or phase, to be passed through and left behind. Instead, he proposes that we not ground it as some "fixed state" but consider, rather, the very experience of the crossing-over, that we insist on it (*Seminar-N* 51/*WS* 61). In the crossing-over, the "sound character of language" is not limited to its acoustic meaning.[12] Heidegger makes an interesting move here: he takes Herder's argument about hearing and reconstructs it so that hearing is no longer acoustic in nature but grounded in attention and a unique mode of relating to the world, thereby establishing the crossing-over as enabling what bears sound as well as what remains silent, both internal and external. This intermediate realm bears on what Heidegger calls "the sensible realm of language" (*sinnlichen Bereich der Sprache*) (*Seminar-T* 156/*WS* 189), which he describes as the realm that allows "the crossing-over from inner to outer word and ascertains the unity of both [stellt die Einheit von beiden fest]. . . . In this manner the unity of the inner and outer word is given since they are both based in sensibility" [in der Sinnlichkeit gründen] (*Seminar-T* 156/*WS* 190).

An accurate account of Heidegger's interpretative move here, requires a new set of terms. Heidegger presents his idea of the crossing-over as an alternative to what he considers to be Herder's deficient account of the possibility of crossing-over from the external to the internal, the sonorous to the nonsonorous. The deficiency in Herder's account is especially notable in the blank, mute space of the in-between, a space on which Heidegger focuses his discussion. Herder provides the proper material, so to speak, but fails to develop a proper account of what Heidegger takes to be the meaning of the *Treatise* "as a whole." The crossing-over is therefore not some external addition to Herder's theory but rather a virtually new formulation of its very components.

Let me first reconstruct the argument from Heidegger's somewhat loose preparatory notes for the seminar, in which he discusses the unique role of the sheep's bleating in the *Treatise*. From the very beginning, Heidegger emphasizes that Herder's preoccupation with the example of the bleating sheep does not focus on its sound character and therefore "cannot be understood in acoustical terms. . . . Rather, the "breaking-free" of the tone [bleating] is to be understood as an advancing towards us, in such a manner that what advances falls behind and comes to stand in itself" (*Seminar-T* 166/*WS* 204). But what does "breaking free" mean here? Heidegger describes the bleating as an "erecting-up" of the sound, a "contrasting-that-lifts-out, contrasting-that-lifts-itself-out" (*Seminar-N* 119–120/*WS* 137). While sticking to acoustic terms (sound, tone, hearing), Heidegger establishes a conceptual configuration that opens up a much wider framework.

This is reflected in one of Heidegger's diagrams:

The inner (drawing in) [*Die innige (einholende)*]	}	Attuned [*gestimmte*]	}	
spreading out [*Ausbreitung*]	}	Insistence [*Inständigkeit*]	}	being-there [*Da*-sein]
The removing gathering [*Die entruckende Sammlung*]	}	in the in-between [*Im Inzwischen*]	}	

(*Seminar-N* 93/*WS* 109)

The diagram traces the movement between the human being and the sounding object—in this case, the bleating sheep. It is through this emphasis on movement that Heidegger establishes that human language for Herder is not at all about speech or the human ear, nor is it about the mere ability to hear and identify sounds. Language is humans' way of being in the world, their movement in and relation to it. "Being attuned" in the second column opens up the possibility to notice the crossing-over or the "in-between." In other words, sound proffers a relationship that is now revealed as decidedly linguistic and emerges only insofar as the human being senses a movement and becomes part of it. It is, therefore, only with the "to" and the "from" of movement that something presents itself as the sounding object—"sound announces its provenance" (*Seminar-T* 159/*WS* 193)—thus allowing the objective presence (of the sheep) to emerge. The reciprocities between humans' attunement toward the world (a movement outward, "from") and the drawing-in and insistence, the forceful penetration of the bleating into the soul (an inner movement, "to"), constitute the origin of language (*Seminar-T* 159/*WS* 193). Considering Heidegger's diagram in light of Herder's *Treatise*, it is important to remember that for Herder the sheep's bleating is but a first step in his account of the emergence of human language. Regardless of the question of whether sound is external or internal, it is the sheep as a linguistic object in which the described process culminates. The human being is attentive to sounds that claim his attention, he then echoes these sounds silently in his soul, eventually being able to notice a *sheep*, not merely its bleating.

The *to-from* pattern of movement appears in the diagram together with the term *gathering*, understood here as a movement of language: man perceives, and thereby turns outward to the bleating sound; this movement is then followed by a second movement of the sound inward, into the soul: a relationship comes into being, and language is what grounds it. Heidegger's reconstruction of Herder's argument illuminates how the movement of reaching out to the world is inextricably tied to the countermovement of letting the world in. Heidegger uses *gathering* here in a double sense: first, the listener's soul *gathers* the bleating sound into an object; and second, as it pays attention to the sheep's bleating, the soul perceives itself in the act of paying attention: "to *gather* oneself in a moment of *wake*, to acknowledge something as differentiated and differentiating in oneself. . . . Ac-knowledgment . . . to perceive ob-ject and thus to perceive *oneself with* it" (*Seminar-N* 17/*WS* 20–21). Paying attention involves precisely this: Besonnenheit establishes man's ability to be attentive, to take notice (*merken*) and attend to (*aufmerken*)—then followed by a demarking (*abmerken*) or making noticeable to oneself (*bemerkbar machen*).[13]

Further on Heidegger elaborates on the relationship between attention and sign formation, writing that "to notice *tones* and to form [them] into *marks*—to convey to the *tongue* through the *ear*" together constitute the possibility of "sounding *out* the inner word" (*Seminar-N* 114/*WS* 132). Heidegger distinguishes here between two distinct features of the resounding of the inner word: (1) the movement itself, "presencing of the di-fference of the from-towards" (2) "that which is moved, itself moving—come toward the one who hears—*Breaking-free* and *yet remaining on*!" (*Seminar-N* 114/*WS* 132). The sheep is now present as a mark within the soul, but this mark appears (and this is crucial) as part of a relationship rather than as a representation of an object. The gathering inherent to language entails that the objects perceived are always already perceived as taking part in a relationship with speaking man. To recall, this is one of the important factors in Rousseau's argument (discussed in chapter 3): the criterion of the accuracy or truth value of the word "giant" is not limited to knowledge of the object but constituted by the relationship the latter has with the speaker (in Rousseau's case, the relation between the savage and the "other [man]").

Heidegger is fascinated by Herder's idea of the "inner word," specifically, with the transformation of the acoustic sense data, first into a characteristic-mark and then an inner word. Perceiving and noticing the object is not the same as constituting it *as* object; to achieve the latter the mark (*Merkmal*) is crucial. As the transcript of the sixth class clearly manifests, it is only due to the mark of the bleating that the sheep can be experienced as a unified "white, soft, woolly" object, "since only now is indeed a substrate won, a starting point for possible experience: precisely the 'one bleating'! The inner mark-word is now to be seen in the mark" [Im Merkmal nun ist das innere Merkwort zu sehen] (*Seminar-T* 150/*WS* 181). The bleating sound breaks free from the sheep, becomes separate and distinct, and is subsequently received by the soul and resounds within it.[14] Heidegger observes, however, that despite the fact that the sound leaves the creature sounding it, Herder does not treat the bleating as an isolated sign or reference mark pointing at a preexisting object (according to Heidegger, doing so would wrongly limit language to being a product of mere abstraction) or as something "self-standing" outside the soul (*Seminar-T* 151, 152/*WS* 182, 183). Instead,

> by the soul receiving this bleating [dies Blöken aufnimmt], by it bleating inside itself, its bleating and the bleating one become one inner thing for it [zum einem Inneren]—and as this inner, as name, as tone, that which is perceived henceforth has its true being [Sein]. Only as an inner *is* the animal for the human being (respectively the thing in general); but just this inner is the human being himself. (*Seminar-T* 152/*WS* 183)

The animal has, perhaps, an objective status outside the sensing, hearing soul, but it can become an object *for the human*, an object of language, only when it resounds in the inner space of the soul. When this sound penetrates the soul, it "does not remain clinging in the ears, not in through one and out the other." Herder's understanding of language is, rather, "a moment in the relational order of the recognition of a being as such" (*Seminar-T* 151/*WS* 183). Words are first and foremost inner words and are therefore not representations of objects, but rather—going back to the diagram with which we started— a "journey into the attunement and mood" [die Fahrt in die Gestimmtheit und Stimmung] of the encounter with the object (*Seminar-N* 128/*WS* 149). Heidegger's emphasis lies elsewhere: for him the sound character of language is not its simple, mere reality. It belongs to a different, essential reality, which serves as the condition for the existence of mere acoustic sound (*Seminar-N* 109/*WS* 128). This argument marks the crucial moment of transition from the merely acoustic meaning of hearing (*Hören*) into an altogether different understanding of hearing as attention and listening (*Hörschen*): hearkening.

In his interpretative move from hearing to hearkening, Heidegger makes the point that although the *Treatise* holds the clues for this transition, they were not placed there intentionally: without properly grasping it and assessing its importance, Herder here performs an interpretation of hearing as *hearkening* in the sense of *being-attentive-on* (*Seminar-N* 101/*WS* 117). Heidegger continues a few sections later: "In spite of all Herder remains with this stress on hearing and hearkening in the "acoustical"-"phonetical." . . . He does not even see the essence of hearing as hearkening and still less the inner connection of hearing *as hearkening with being attentive* (reflective awareness, perceiving); he does not realize that he sees the "sense of hearing" already *essentially* different" (*Seminar-N* 108/*WS* 128). This claim is disputable (in chapter 3 I have shown precisely this point to the effect that Herder was in fact aware of the difference), but Heidegger insists on maintaining his critical, sometimes scornful tone regarding Herder's *Treatise* throughout the *Seminar*. At times this may appear as an attempt to claim one of Herder's central ideas as his own. The importance of Heidegger's analysis is that he does not *replace* hearing with hearkening but rather gives account of the attentive aspect of hearing. When we hear, we not only register the sounds around us; we also, and here foremost, engage in a relationship with our surroundings: we are oriented within it; we experience our relations with other beings and with our selves. This is why, for Heidegger, listening to the sheep's bleating is not at all about the sound: "bahh"; it has to do with our ability to sense ourselves in relation to the bleating sheep, to the way it "erects" or arises before us by way of its sounding. Heidegger foregrounds this in one of his seminar notes when he writes: the fact that "here the sense of hearing as perceiving with the ear has in no way priority" demonstrates that "it is grasped as perceiving in the sense of being-attentive, of hearkening, of being-silent" (*Seminar-N* 105/*WS* 123). That is, perceived *sounds* have no priority over the internal, nonsounding ones (*Seminar-N* 107/*WS* 125).[15] Heidegger then poses the following question: "Does the human being hearken because he can hear, or can *he hear* because he can hearken? And what does *being able to hearken* mean? And *what* does the human being "hear"? That to which he *hearkens—what does he hearken to?*" (*Seminar-N* 94/*WS* 110).

Hearing and Hearkening

Heidegger's exposition of the crossing-over as a response to the difficulties posed by the *Treatise* remains, however, rather obscure, or at least, somewhat schematic. Reading the *Seminar*, one has the sense that while the crucial problems are indeed sketched out and the crossing-over seems to be an appropriate idea with which to tackle them there is nevertheless no full realization and development of this solution. To fully comprehend this argument, recourse to other writings by Heidegger is important. Although the question of hearing appears here in the context of his discussion of Herder, Heidegger was preoccupied with similar questions throughout his career, starting more than a decade earlier, especially in the context of his ongoing interpretation of Heraclitus' fragments; this discussion begins in the mid-1930s and continues well into the late 1960s. I refer to his 1935 *Introduction to Metaphysics* whose last chapter is devoted to a discussion of *Logos* and Being in Heraclitus;[16] "Logos: Heraclitus B50" (1951);[17] the fifth of the *Freiburg Lectures* (1957);[18] and finally, *Heraclitus*, a seminar devoted to Heraclitus that Heidegger taught together with Eugene Fink in 1966–67.[19] I revisit these texts in order to enrich his remarks on Herder in the *Seminar*, which touch on surprisingly similar issues. My discussion of hearing, hearkening, and gathering will therefore move freely between the *Seminar* and Heidegger's aforementioned works.

The consideration of hearing, hearkening, and gathering appears in the context of Heidegger's exploration of Heraclitus and the meaning of λόγος (*logos*). In search of the origin of the term, before Western thought secured its signification as "speech," Heidegger resorts to Heraclitus. In his reading of Heraclitus' first two fragments, he shows that for the Greeks, *logos*, rather than referring to mere speech, word, or doctrine, was originally associated with a group of terms related to the verb "to gather" so that "everything that happens, that is, that comes into being, stands there in accordance with this constant Together" (*IM* 135 [98]). Reflecting on the history of logos, Heidegger shows that the term originates from the word *légein*, that means to say or tell, as well as to gather or collect. Logos, in other words, is not simply speech or a word, but rather an activity that has to do with different forms of gathering and collecting. For Heraclitus, logos as gathering is therefore not a merely a sound expression of some preexistent idea or concept but a way of gathering, bringing into a unity.[20] This is where hearing enters the discussion. Heidegger refers to several of Heraclitus' Fragments, but 50B is his focal point: "So long as we only listen to the sound of the word as the expression of the speaker, we are not listening at all" (Heidegger's translation). In his reading of the fragment, Heidegger links between "hearing" as it is used by Heraclitus, and "gathering" or "attending." Heidegger introduces an important difference between "hearing" and "hearkening," as mentioned, two central terms in the *Seminar*.[21]

Drawing on Heraclitus, Heidegger distinguishes between hearing and hearkening, arguing that the anatomical and physiological elements of everyday acoustic hearing are not the central ones, since these

> never bring about a hearing, not even if we take this solely as an apprehending of noises, sounds, and tones. . . . So long as we think of hearing along the lines of acoustical science, everything is made to stand on its head. We wrongly think that the activation of the body's audio equipment is hearing proper. (*Logos* 65)

Acoustic hearing has therefore a quality of deafness: the more open the ear to the acoustic aspect of discourse and dialogue, the more it undermines our ability to grasp, understand, and *hearken*. Heidegger's claim seems counterintuitive at first: instead of linking between the sense of hearing and awareness of the presence of things, he argues that it is precisely due to our sense of hearing, which we feel connects us to our surrounding world, that we become absent from it, or present-absent. Mere hearing, he writes in *IM*, "strews and scatters itself" in *doxa* or seeming, so that those who merely hear can perhaps hear words and discourse, "yet they are closed off to what they should listen to." Closely following Heraclitus' Fragment 34, Heidegger describes them as "hearers who resemble the deaf," "those who are absently present," dwelling "in the midst of things, and yet they are away" (*IM* 137 [99]).[22]

Hearkening, on the other hand, which is closer to Heraclitus' logos, is independent of mouth or ear and refers to attending and being attentive. According to his reading of Fragment 50, and in very similar terms to those he uses in the *Seminar*, Heidegger argues that genuine hearkening has nothing to do with the ear or tongue. We can only hear when we already hearken (*IM* 136 [99]). This is why the reference to "ear lobes and eardrums" (*Ohrläppchen und Trommelfelle*) as the organs of hearing, is merely accidental (*HT* 267 [368–369]). On account of these distinctions, Heidegger formulates Heraclitus' argument as follows: "Human beings do hear, and they hear words, but in this hearing they cannot 'hearken' to—that is, follow—what is not audible like words, what is not *talk* but *logos*. . . . Correspondingly, genuine hearing as Being-obedient is opposed to mere hearing and keeping one's ears open" (*IM* 136–137 [99]). It is the former (hearkening) that makes the latter (hearing) possible, that grounds it. Heidegger returns to this idea almost thirty years later in the above-mentioned joint seminar he taught together with Eugen Fink. In a dialogue between them on the relationship between vision and hearing, Heidegger remarks, "In the dark I see nothing, and nevertheless I see" (*Heraclitus* 128). To this, Fink responds with an elaborate account of the sense of hearing:

> This is similar with hearing. A sentry, for instance, listens intensely into the silence without hearing something determinate. *When he hears no determinate sound, still he hears.* His hearkening is the most intense wakefulness of wanting to hear. *Harkening is the condition of possibility for hearing.* It is being open to the space of the hearable, whereas hearing is meeting the specifically hearable. (*Heraclitus* 128, my italics)

Fink's argument ties the threads together: we are usually preoccupied with our ability to hear, in the acoustical, everyday context. The implications of this focus on hearing, however, have made us deaf to hearkening. To cite Matthew Meyer, it is in "the banal familiarity of our encountering the 'hearable' we have lost our ability to listen for something deeper than or beyond mere determinations of words. That is to say, by hearing all of the time, we have lost our ability to listen, even to open up to the possibility of listening."[23] We can be incapable of hearkening and thereby withheld from logos, understood in its original meaning as *légein,* namely, laying forth and gathering, regardless of our ability to hear sounds with our ears (*IM* 137). We have lost our ability to pay attention, to gather and be gathered. We hear, yet we don't pay attention; we are immersed in sound and thereby become deaf to silence. But, Fink explains, insofar as we can see in the dark, we can also hearken when no sound is heard. In hearing we adhere to "something determined," hearable; whereas in hearkening we are attuned, attentive, open to the possibility of the *hearable* (*Heraclitus* 128).[24]

Returning to the *Seminar,* Heidegger argues that what is heard (*Das Gehörte*) can only be audible if it is already *hearkened to* (*Erhorchtes*); at the same time, however, the acoustic tone urges the *hearkened to* (*Erhorchtes*). Heidegger uses the expression *Ohrenspitzen* here, suggesting a sharpened, attentive mode of hearing. Hearkening is therefore not limited to the acoustic perception of sound but more essentially, as Heidegger writes, to the "fore-having [Vor-habe] and fore-taking [Vor-nahme] of what essences-on [An-wesendem], essences-to" [Zu-wesendem] (*Seminar-N* 120/*WS* 138). The human being *hears* the sound of the bleating; but more than anything, he hearkens. He notices and is attentive to it and perceives it insofar as he is open to it; this is an *openness for,* that is "simultaneously withdrawing and yet leaving what is taken in its place—yes indeed—*going beyond sound and tone*" (*Seminar-N* 93/*WS* 109). The quintessence of hearkening in Heidegger's reading of Herder is exemplified in the following assertion: "Attention grounds in hearkening, but hearkening the deeper essence of reason" [Das Merken gründet im Horchen, aber das Horchen das tiefere Wesen der Vernunft] (*Seminar-N* 119/*WS* 137). After devoting numerous pages of the *Seminar* to his fierce criticism of Herder's emphasis on reason, he replaces it here with what he himself considers the essence of the human being: hearkening.

Here Heidegger resorts to the notion of *gathering* (*Sammlung*). The term appears throughout the *Seminar* in the context of his account of hearing and should be addressed against the background of his preceding discussion of Heraclitus and the relationship between logos and légein, language and gathering. According to Heidegger, the centrality of hearing for Herder is not limited to a mere form of receptivity; hearing is, rather, a decidedly active sense and has to do with the human ability to *gather*: when man hears he gathers the heard object, and at the same time gathers himself, is collected in his attention to sound. Hearing is a "*spreading out to . . . removing to . . .* and this simultaneously with the *receiving* and *collecting,* with the in-nerness (taking within into the inner) as a gathering, holding in . . . *inner spreading out and gathering that removes,* no more dispersion and scattering . . . rather: *mediating* middle, that *goes for* the middle and at the same time always *swings out*" (*Seminar-N* 102/*WS* 119). It is interesting to compare these remarks with Heidegger's account of the relationship between saying and gathering in *Basic Principles of Thinking* (his 1957 Freiburg lectures).

In the context of his discussion of saying, Heidegger argues that every form of speaking is necessarily a "saying"; however, saying does not mean speaking in the sense of a utilization of our speech organs. Saying is rather "a bringing as a bringing-to, which at the same time brings us away from here and brings us into what is said. The gentle power (*Gewalt*) of a bringing pervades saying."[25] It is fascinating to compare this with the *Seminar* where Heidegger repeats in similar words: "In language we gather objects in such a way that this gathering is at the same time a saying. But this gathering that is contained in language is what we mean when we say 'thinking.' Language is therefore understood doubly, it is thinking and in saying" (*Seminar-T* 133/*WS* 156). Considered together with the former, these remarks illustrate Heidegger's accentuation of the kinship between the outward movement of spreading and reaching out, and the opposite inwardly directed movement of reception by way of withdrawal. These two contradictory movements constitute, in effect, the condition of the formation of an intermediate space, an in-between-ness, that allows the gathering. Crossing-over and gathering appear therefore in tandem.[26]

Heidegger continues with an interesting move: he explains attention by establishing a link between hearing (*hören*), the sense of hearing (*Gehör*), and belonging (*Gehören*). In gathering we constitute a relationship to what is heard, we make it our own. Heidegger explains:

> Mortals hear the thunder of the heavens, the rustling of woods, the gurgling of fountains, the ringing of plucked strings, the rumbling of motors, the noises of the city—only and only so far as they always already in some way *belong to them and yet do not belong to them*. . . .[W]hen does hearing succeed? *We have heard* [gehört] *when we belong to* [gehören] *matter addressed.* (*Logos* 65–66, my emphasis)[27]

To take these remarks back to the *Seminar* and the diagram cited above, the "breaking free" of the bleating tone initiates a twofold movement: a "toward me," and a turning of me toward. With these two movements, "a distinction comes to presence. . . .[I]t is precisely in the movement that what is noticeable becomes noticeable." When the human being hears the bleating, the sound enters his soul, seizes it, making it *belong*. The sheep is now not merely an object that produces sounds but inseparable from the human soul. At this moment of encounter between sound and soul, "the thus encountered human being says 'you' " (*Seminar-T* 159/*WS* 193). This interpretation of Herder is clarified by reference to *Logos*. The moment of relation, of belonging, is that of the in-between: when the sheep belongs, and not yet belongs, to the one listening to it. The human being is attentive, open to the bleating that penetrates the soul—but this moment of passage can only occur when the relation is being constituted in the not-yet.

To recall, Heidegger criticizes Herder for his disjoint, fissured description of the human being. The sense of hearing brought together with gathering provides Heidegger with a potential resolution: together they form an in-between space structured on the basis of the sense of hearing that Heidegger characterizes as a "sensorium commune . . . a gathering, unifying sense. . . . Thus the sense of hearing is in Herder the place where all feelings come together, where the making-present of the sensible world is originally executed" (*Seminar-T* 155/ *WS* 188)[28]—a coalescent human being emerges from the sense of hearing, and hearing is the foundation of language.

The Silence of Language

Heidegger's use of the idea of the crossing-over in response to the conspicuous breaches in Herder's argument leads him to develop the conception of a nonsonorous (or, not merely acoustic) language. The earlier mentioned discussion of hearing and hearkening bears this out, where the latter is shown to be a more primary and fundamental form of linguistic relation, based not only on sound or the sense of hearing but also on silent attention and taking notice. In my interpretation of Heidegger so far, I have concentrated on the latter, yet it remains to be seen what it means to speak silently, to express without uttering a word, and finally, how (if at all) one can hear and respond to such silent linguistic expressions. When Heidegger poses the question, "Language characterizes the human being—but who is the human being?" [aber wer ist der Mensch?] (*Seminar-N* 39/*WS* 48), he is in fact asking whether human beings may be linguistic creatures without uttering a word or taking in any sound.

Before I address this question, let me emphasize that although Heidegger's ideas feature as a critical alternative to Herder, we have already seen in the previous chapters that the *Treatise* actually offers some very explicit statements that clearly imply the idea of a nonacoustic language. This is especially evident in Herder's discussion of the "inner word of the soul." Human language is not a cry of sensations, he writes, not based on imitation, and it also does not originate from communication or propositional expressions: it is Besonnenheit, attention, orientation. This then enables Herder to argue that "even a blind and dumb man, one sees, would inevitably invent language, if only he is not without feeling and deaf" (*Treatise* 98/*AS* 735) and "even the person who was dumb all his life, if he was a human being, if he took awareness, had language in his soul!" (*Treatise* 90/*AS* 725). Language emerges, then, as what Herder calls "the common-understanding of his soul with itself, and a common-understanding as necessary as the human being was human being" [Einverständnis seiner Seele mit sich und ein so notwendiges Einverständnis, als der Mensch Mensch war] (*Treatise* 90/

AS 725). Let me use this last sentence to turn back to Heidegger's corresponding account of the silent call of conscience in *Being and Time*'s Division II.

The call of conscience (*Gewissen*) is as an internal voice in which and with which Dasein calls and responds to itself, thereby disclosing itself to itself as Dasein. Heidegger evokes the idea in *Being and Time* in the context of his discussion of the authentic potentiality of Dasein, a potentiality numbed or lost due to Dasein's immersion within "the they" (*Das Mann*): "Because Da-sein is lost in the 'they,' it must first *find* itself. In order to find *itself* at all, it must be 'shown' to itself in its possible authenticity" (*BT* 248 [268]). In the context of our discussion here, Heidegger describes Dasein's being lost and found again in acoustic terms. Immersed within the sounds of everyday chatter or discourse, Dasein has lost its ability to listen to itself as well as the unique kind of hearing that is required for such listening. The call of conscience embodies the authentic voicing and listening Heidegger is after, but in a wholly nonsonorous configuration. Heidegger characterizes the call of conscience by contrasting it with everyday discourse and communication. Discourse consists of the communication of information *about* something; it has a propositional, intentional structure and is established on a correspondence between speaker and addressee. The call of conscience, on the other hand, does not communicate any information, it says nothing and has nothing to tell; it "is lacking any kind of utterance. It does not even come to words, and yet it is not at all obscure and indefinite" (*BT* 252 [273]).

In his "Heidegger's Ear," Derrida is preoccupied with the central role hearing plays in Heidegger, especially regarding the idea of the implications of hearing a voice that does not speak. This voice, he writes, is not to be understood as an acoustic phenomenon and, accordingly, does not assume the ear to be an organ listening to some external utterance. Discussing Heidegger's claims in *Being and Time*, Derrida writes of hearing that it is "constitutive of discourse, but does not consist in an acoustic phenomenon of the physiopsychological order; hearing has no need of the 'inner' or the 'outer,' that is, the ear in the organic sense of the word."[29] Derrida takes on Heidegger's "voice of a friend" which is carried by Dasein[30] as the starting point of his essay:

> The voice of this friend does not necessarily speak. . . . Through its voice that I hear, I hear the friend itself, beyond its voice but in that voice. I hear and carry the friend with me in hearing its voice. . . . Dasein "carries" the friend itself, but not the friend in its totality, in flesh and blood. Dasein carries it, one might say, in the figure of the voice, its metonymic figure (a part for the whole).[31]

For Derrida this "carrying" (*Tragen*) is the key to understanding the possibility of hearing what is not said, what is not external in any way to Dasein or to the ear. Dasein hears a voice it carries with it, neither inside, nor outside, but within. What matters is not the said or saying of the said, but rather the hearing (*das Hören*) of its voice.[32]

Characterizing the call as a vague, indefinite expression (which ushers in the risk of being interpreted as mere nonsense) does not weaken the call of conscience, on the contrary. According to Heidegger, it is precisely its nonpropositional and nonsonorous nature that grants the call of conscience its power to summon (*Anruf*) Dasein, to call it back from the idle talk of the everyday. But this requires, obviously, a great deal of effort. Dasein is surrounded by the endless, empty sounds of "the they," sounds similar to what Heidegger referred to in his already mentioned reading of Heraclitus. To be able to listen to itself Dasein must be impervious to these sounds; Dasein must develop *deafness* in order to *hear*. The call of conscience is therefore not the negation of speech or everyday language; it opens, rather, the possibility to hear the silence, to listen to what has nothing to say, yet calls us forth ever more powerfully (*BT* 253 [274]). Heidegger thus repeatedly mentions that in order for Dasein to be able to call and listen to itself, there has to be a certain form of disruption or break with its listening to everyday idle talk, from which it needs to be *called back*. As Brogan puts it: "This special call of self to itself is a kind of jolting of everydayness and the stupor of absorption and evasion. But this rupture or rift (*Bruch*) is a modality of Dasein's being. That means in a sense that all communication and idle talk, all everydayness, is haunted by this disruption, at least as an existential possibility."[33] This haunting is crucial: Heidegger is not interested only in the possibility of listening to the call but foregrounds the presence of impossibility, of a hearing (of idle talk) that is forever haunted by its own disintegration, that serves in turn as the condition for a different kind of listening (to oneself). Put differently, this is the inauthentic that is always haunted by the authentic.[34]

It is only in a silent voice that Dasein can address itself: it is a unique form of address, one that has nothing to say, is inherently silent: "Conscience speaks solely and constantly in the mode of silence" [Schweigen] (*BT* 252 [273]). The call is silent because it calls only the one summoned (and is called by him), and furthermore, it calls him and her not from within the public, idle chatter of "the they," but rather, "*calls* him *back* from that *to the reticence of his existent potentiality-of-being*" (*BT* 256 [277]). Heidegger is at his peak here insofar as the unique vocabulary of *Being and Time* is concerned; however, the idea of the silent call of conscience, and especially Dasein's ability to recognize and respond to it, is distinctly similar to the preceding discussion of hearing, hearkening, and gathering. Here too, listening to one's own call requires a special kind of attention, one that will allow Dasein to suppress its *hearing* of the sounds of the everyday, so as to be able to *hearken* to its own internal, silent call. Brogan's interpretation of this break from the numbing effect of idle talk is important here. He argues that the call of conscience should not be understood as the mere opposite of communicative, propositional language. Conscience is, in fact, the condition of communication; it is the "coming together of facticity and existence." Understood this way, Heidegger touches on the possibility to hear and respond to the call, not instead of idle discourse but, rather, from within it.[35]

Heidegger suggests a unique kind of intensive, attentive hearing, that is to say, hearkening. Just as in his reading of Heraclitus, the silent *voice* of the call as well as the ability to hearken to it do not occur, essentially, in ordinary discourse. The call is not external in any way—it neither comes from the outside nor is heard as a call *entering* Dasein's internal realm, nor does it result in any form of externalization of inner content transmitted to an addressee. It emerges and transpires thoroughly within. As opposed to the structure of discourse or propositional expressions, in which an utterance is spoken out, refers to something, and is communicated to someone—in the call of conscience this structure collapses into itself. What is talked about—the one calling and the one summoned by the call—are all one and the same thing: Dasein itself.

Heidegger separates here between what he calls the self, and the they-self. The latter disintegrates when the former takes the stage: "Because only the *self* of the they-self is summoned and made to hear, the *they* collapses" (*BT* 252 [273]). Despite the indefinite, even vague definition of the call's context and communicative structure, Heidegger makes it very clear that the call cannot be overlooked by Dasein because what it discloses is unequivocal; it is starkly clear in its address and summoning. "'Deceptions' occur in conscience not by an oversight of the call (a mis-calling) but only because the call is *heard* in such a way that, instead of being understood authentically, it is drawn by the they-self into a manipulative conversation with one's self and is distorted in its character of disclosure" (*BT* 253 [274]). This account not only accentuates the nonsonorous linguistic form of communication with oneself, but, with the introduction of the unequivocalness of the summoning, it resituates the whole discussion in the moral sphere.

The structure of the call of conscience seems, then, to largely correspond to Herder's understanding of language: the soul speaks to itself; the human being is a creature of language regardless of having a mouth or ears, and finally, summoning (as well as gathering), which seems very close to Herder's understanding of attention and awareness. Herder and Heidegger share a conception of language that is not limited to propositional utterances or communication. These similarities, however, do not tell the whole story. The emergence of the call of conscience marks the moment in which language, understood as discourse, collapses into itself, creating an intermediary space in which Dasein stands before itself. Although Herder too speaks of an inner space and inner word in humans, his account continues with a discussion of how this internal movement of language may revert outward. Heidegger's silent, summoning call remains internal and continues to resound in the solipsistic inner space of Dasein. The authenticity of the call (insofar as authenticity is the opposite of Heidegger's use of "deception" in the above quote) is also established internally, when Dasein recognizes its own call to itself from the idle sounds of the everyday, to let it "erect up," appear as a singular point of gathering, and to hearken to it.

The call of conscience serves Heidegger well in his attempt to set forth the different ways in which Dasein can encounter or reencounter itself, call itself back from its immersion in idle chatter and the *they*. Conscience is, in Heidegger's account, an opening of Dasein to itself, a potentiality. But, significantly, the call can serve as potential only within the horizons opened by Heidegger in the first place. When it hearkens to the call, Dasein discloses its innermost being, its array of possibilities, while leaving language behind. The move performed in *Being and Time*'s sections on the call of conscience begins with a nonsonorous conception of language that is very much in line with Heidegger's interest in the *Seminar*. In the context of his project in *Being and Time*, however, recourse to the silent call and the ability to hearken to silence is not made with the aim of rethinking the structure of language but rather concerns questions of authenticity and being. My own interest in Herder's conception of language lies elsewhere: his focus on the nonsonorous, on attention and gathering, is important insofar as it puts language at the center of the discussion, offering us a way to extend and enrich its conceptualization instead of leaving it behind.

Another perspective on the limitations of Heidegger's account of conscience emerges when we take the relationship between Herder's two languages into account. Although the nonsonorous, silent language of Besonnenheit in the *Treatise* is neither limited to mere speech or communication nor defined by its imparting of information or turning to an addressee, Herder's account does not entail an enclosed, solipsistic structure. On the contrary, the description of the primary language of pain and sensations culminates in the very strong postulation of a sympathetic community:

> Now let it not be touched, this weak, sensitive being! As alone and individual and exposed to every hostile storm of the universe as it seems, it is not alone; it stands allied [im Bunde] with the whole of nature!, delicately strung, but nature has hidden in these strings sounds which, stimulated and encouraged, awaken other equally delicately built creatures in turn, and can communicate sparks [Funken] to a remote heart, as though through an invisible chain, so that it feels for this unseen creature. (*Treatise* 66/*AS* 698)[36]

Heidegger's conception of the call of conscience suggests a solipsistic sphere conditioned by Dasein's break away from the discourse with others, problematizing the moral significance of conscience. Herder presents a different picture in which the centrality of the inner word and the soul speaking to itself does not exclude the possibility of sympathy and *Mitsein*. This precisely is the core of Herder's conception of language: expressibility and shareability do not depend on the propositional or communicative nature of language. Thus, pain returns to the foreground.

A Final Remark on Pain

Despite its internal incongruities—its forceful expressive nature together with its fundamental privacy and unshareability—we have already seen that the experience of pain has a strong, stable core. Regardless of the direction of its expression, outward or inward, pain is distinguished by the immediacy with which it becomes almost identical to us, those who bear it. To put it slightly differently, pain's power lies not in its ability to destroy our bodies or identities (as Scarry would have it) but in its incomparable capacity to occupy our attention. Such attentiveness, however, does not mean—and therein lies my point—that we become wholly enclosed within our suffering bodies or souls, that we completely lose all connection to the world, to others. Pain's overwhelming demand, rather, implies its ability to capture our attention so violently that we have no choice but to attend to it. C. S. Lewis writes that "Pain insists upon being attended to. God whispers to us in our pleasures, speaks in our consciences, but shouts in our pains. It is his megaphone to rouse a deaf world."[37] Here the issue is neither isolation nor destructiveness but rather our unresponsiveness to suffering, which God faces by shouting in our pains which becomes a megaphone of attention. This manifests itself first insofar as our attention and relationship to ourselves changes, yet it has the power to radically affect our relationship to the world too. As for the latter, the far-reaching, startling implications that pain has for our experience of the world and our relationship to others emerge not when the latter are changed *because* of our pain (others do not understand us, are not sympathetic to our suffering, etc.) but because our own attention to and orientation in the world radically change. Our body, which is and was always there, unreflected and unnoticed, suddenly becomes the center of our existence, and everything else revolves around it,[38] but it is not the only thing present. Pain becomes our yardstick.[39]

But there is more to it: pain's way of monopolizing our attention has to do with its concomitance. Pain reveals itself to us but equally allows us to face ourselves—both with an unmatched ferocity. In other cases, when our attention is drawn by something, we are captured by it and lose ourselves in it. In pain, however, we not only "have" pain or are concentrated on it as though it were some kind of an object we possessed; rather, as I mentioned earlier, we *become* pain, so that in our heightened state of attention to it, we are, in fact, attentive to our very selves. To use Jean-Luc Marion's wonderful description:

> As soon as I suffer, I suffer myself . . . as soon as I suffer it is in, by, and from myself that I suffer. The iron and the fire inasmuch as suffered no longer appear to the world, but appear in myself. . . . I suffer *myself* by them. Between the iron and the fire and me who suffers them, the gap disappears. I can no longer make a retreat into a more withdrawn tower: once the enclosure has been invested, I am definitively invaded, taken, done. Suffering rivets me to myself as one rivets something to the ground—by earthing. Suffering does not only hurt me, it assigns me especially to myself as flesh.[40]

I suggest we understand this "assigning me to myself" in terms of attention. Returning to the *Treatise*, let us take another look at Herder's account of Besonnenheit, and specifically, his thought-provoking description of the human ability to pay attention. To recall, Herder describes "an ocean of sensations" flooding the human soul, which in turn, becomes immersed in, and overwhelmed by it. This is where Besonnenheit and reflection enter, as a force of the soul that enables it to "separate off [absondern], stop, and pay attention [Aufmerksamkeit] to a single wave" (*Treatise* 87/*AS* 722). By way of Besonnenheit, the human being "collects himself" and is able to isolate a single wave—or in Herder's example, the sheep's bleating—and be attentive to it. But this "wave," or sound wave if you will, is not transformed into an object that later becomes the content of man's linguistic expression. Herder suggests a more complex structure here. Paying attention to a single wave essentially refers to the human capacity to take in the world, to attend to it differently, although it was always already there. In other words, attention is about a movement of return, a re-turning to what was always already there. But Besonnenheit is not only about attention; it also registers the ability to reflect and be conscious of man's own attentiveness (*Treatise* 87/*AS* 722). Man withdraws from the flood, takes a step back and notices the wave; but at the same time, he is also capable of noticing his own act of attention, in other words, he is reflective. Herder comments on the difference between the singling out of an external object in the flood (bleating, for instance) and the ability to reflect on one's own capacity of attention as such (*Treatise* 87/*AS* 722). But what Herder considers in this section is not only the uniqueness of human attention but also and foremost human language. As I already explained in detail,[41] Herder's Besonnenheit, rather than standing for a prelinguistic content, either grants the human being linguistic abilities or is, as it were, indistinguishable from them.

This twofold function of Besonnenheit, as attention and reflection, can be understood in terms of movement: reaching out and being pulled back in are both part of the same motion of collection, reflection and attention. This duality and its productiveness are not only reflected in the two parts of the *Treatise* but also in the structure of pain as such. Pain too is singled out by its expressive movement outward as well as by the intensity with which it pulls us in and encircles us;[42] it cries out while simultaneously being a silent concentration; it is a desperate turn to others and yet there is nothing more private than the experience of pain.

Herder's theory of language demonstrates a singular ability to retain pain's paradoxes as well as to express its inherent connection to language, and this, specifically, by way of the unique interconnection between the language of sensation and human language. Heidegger, however, makes an important contribution: he introduces the term "crossing-over" and insists that Herder's argument can be fully grasped only when the *Treatise* is taken as whole, that is, not split into two languages, human and animal, sound or silence. Using Heidegger's terms in the *Seminar* we could say that the crossing-over allows for a gathering.

Heidegger's importance for an understanding of Herder is, nevertheless, as we have already seen, not exhausted in his explicit discussion of the latter. By way of a concluding remark, therefore, let me point briefly to an important passage in his "Language" where Heidegger provides an illuminating consideration of pain. In the context of his discussion of Georg Trakl's poetry, Heidegger remarks that it would be a mistake to imagine pain as a mere sensation of suffering or affliction.[43] The intimacy inherent to pain should not be thought of psychologically and "as the sort in which sentimentality makes a nest for itself."[44] Heidegger is after a different conception in which instead of an interiority, pain is conceived in terms of intimacy (*Innigkeit*), thereby forming the grounds of our ability to form a relationship. Rather than considering it a mere bodily sensation, thinking of pain as a form of intimacy renders it an essential ground of being in a relation. Heidegger continues:

> But what is pain? Pain rends. It is the rift. But it does not tear apart into dispersive fragments. Pain indeed tears asunder, it separates, yet so that at the same time it draws everything to itself, gathers it to itself. Its rending, as a separating that gathers, is at the same time that drawing which, like the pen-drawing of a plan or sketch, draws and joins together what is held apart in separation. Pain is the joining agent in the rending that divides and gathers. Pain is the joining of the rift. The joining is the threshold. It settles the between, the middle of the two that are separated in it. Pain joins the rift of the difference. Pain is the dif-ference itself.[45]

The importance of Heidegger's claim here lies in that it brings together pain's violent act of separation or "rending" with its unmatched ability to gather. While it no doubt tears us apart (body and soul), this violence comes with pain's inherent capacity to bring us into relationship, supplies the condition of possibility of relation. This is what Heidegger calls the "contrary essence" of pain (*On the Way to Language* 180). Mitchell offers a profound explanation when he writes that

> pain is a wound of relation, and insofar as the tear of pain joins us to the world, this pain is always a shared pain. The discontinuities of pain bring us into continuity with the world. . . . [U]ltimately it is pain that first opens the medial space for this relationality, spilling us into this world *between* subject and object.[46]

It is here that the problematic inherent to the utter closure and solipsism of Heidegger's call of conscience is addressed. Pain is an opening, a potential, a movement of Dasein *back to* itself (in the language of *Being and Time*), and an opening insofar as the structure of language is concerned (to put it in terms of Heidegger's later works). Here Heidegger suggests that understanding pain as rift as well as gathering is inherent to its function as threshold, its liminality: in joining the rift, pain emerges as threshold, as a settling of the in-between, "the middle of the two that are separated in it." A similar idea appears in the context of Heidegger's reading of Trakl's poem "Winter Evening," in which fracture, interruption, and absence function as "thresholds" and pain has "turned the threshold into stone," a phrase Trakl repeats several times. According to Peter Hanly, "It is in and *as* pain that the threshold emerges, becomes possible—that it is "made stone." . . . [P]ain carries the ambivalence, the play, the togetherness of joy and sadness. It is the between space that holds opposites in proximity to one another."[47]

Reconsidered with reference to Herder, pain is a rift that is, essentially, all about the forming of a relationship to a world; it is a way of gathering. The violent, crushing entrance of the bleating sound into the exposed soul, on which it is nothing less than forced, gives birth to the human being's ability to gather and be gathered around it with his inner word of the soul. In his 1955 letter to Ernst Jünger, Heidegger suggests a similar structure when he points at the affinity between the Greek logos (language) and *algos* (pain): "*algos* is related to *alego* which, as an intensive of *lego* signifies intimate gathering [innige Versammlung]. Then pain would be the most intimate of gatherings."[48]

5

Pain, Expression, and Sympathy

Philoctetes

The Figure of Philoctetes

The story of Philoctetes has accompanied major parts of my discussion from the very beginning.[1] As we have seen, Herder was preoccupied with this figure already in his *First Grove* (1769), where he discusses the suffering hero at length in the context of his criticism of Lessing (*First Grove* 72–81). Philoctetes is then briefly mentioned in the *Treatise* (1772: *Treatise* 65/*AS* 697) as an example of the animal's cry of pain as well as in the context of a discussion of sympathy (*Treatise* 140/*AS* 784).[2] But Philoctetes is not only significant insofar as Herder's texts on language and aesthetics are concerned; his presence serves, in more than one way, as a backbone to my arguments regarding the relationship between pain and language. More importantly, it also challenges the two currently presiding theoretical paradigms in the literature about pain with which I began this book.

To recall, according to the first paradigm, pain is destructive not only to our body and mind; it also violently attacks our linguistic capabilities, robbing us of what we consider to be our very humanity. In the second paradigm, as it shatters our language, depriving us of the possibility of communicating, pain destroys every possibility of relating to others, opening an unbridgeable gap between sufferer and world. Pain is thus both destructive and isolating, the first paradigm feeding into the second. I referred to Elaine Scarry's work on pain as exemplary of these two paradigms. Interestingly, Scarry uses Philoctetes' story as representative for her argument regarding pain's unshareability. Referring to Sophocles' play, *Philoctetes*, she describes the dissolution of the boundary between internal and external, arguing how it testifies to an obscene conflation of private and public. Consigned to pain's utter, absolute privacy, Philoctetes is hopelessly enclosed within the solipsistic inexpressibility of his suffering, yet at the same time, he is denied the safety and protection expected from such isolation. Scarry describes this destructive combination as what is experienced spatially claiming that pain either contracts the universe "down to the immediate vicinity of the body" or is experienced as the body swelling to fill the entire universe."[3]

But what is more important in the context of our discussion is the way in which Philoctetes' pain and his shattered language open up, to use Scarry's vocabulary, an absolute split between him and the rest of the world. As the referential structure and function of language disappear, the stark incongruence between the sufferer and the possibility of the empathy of others emerges. Those affected by pain grasp and know it without the slightest doubt; the feeling of pain, to them, is as evident as can be. The opposite is true of those witnessing it from the other side of the abyss: for them, the most immediate, even instinctual experience, as Scarry claims, is their fundamental doubt, to the point of a sense of unreality, of the other's pain.[4] This variance is evinced ten years before the beginning of Sophocles' play, when Philoctetes' peers and soldiers cannot bear the sight and stench of his wound, and are revolted by his uncontrollable screams and swearing. Philoctetes' inarticulate, animal-like cries stir a terrible fear in them, leading them eventually to abandon him for ten long years on the desert island.

The temptation to interpret the story as demonstrating these two paradigms is clear: Philoctetes indeed embodies great suffering—from his wounded, agonizing foot to the pain of betrayal and abandonment. His solitude on the desert island only reinforces his agony and his unremitting cries of pain are a compelling manifestation of that. As the two paradigms would lead us to expect, Philoctetes is destroyed by his pain (body and soul) and his language slowly crumbles into mere cries and exclamations. We could account for this degradation, indeed this loss, of articulate language, by regarding it as instinctive and animal-like, completely outside the bounds of human communication. In this view Philoctetes is violently robbed of these faculties, at the moment when pain "overcomes" language, defeats and silences it, depriving him of his humanity. These two conceptions seem to be present throughout the story, especially around the middle of the play, when Philoctetes experiences a spasm of intense pain that violently robs him of his speech, reducing it to mere exclamations such as "Ah, ah, ah, ah!" and "A-a-a-a-h," until he loses consciousness and collapses. My interpretation of Philoctetes' story and specifically the scene in which the spasm of pain literally strikes him down, is different. The pain-attack scene, in my reading, challenges the two paradigms and bears out that pain is neither merely destructive (of body or of language) nor eventually isolating.

In this chapter, I show that although it may seem so at first, Sophocles' pain-attack scene does not suggest that pain constitutes the impossibility of sympathy, creating a breach between sufferer and witness. Instead, when Philoctetes, attacked by the spasm of pain, can only stammer and cry out, he is not deprived of language but rather endowed with one, however inarticulate or nonpropositional. Furthermore, when Neoptolemus witnesses Philoctetes' extreme pain and his own petrified response to it, he is only hesitant at first; later, however, he neither withdraws nor abandons—quite the opposite. Instead of violently opening up a breach between the two, the expressions of pain institute a unique space of intimacy between the one in pain and the one who witnesses it. It is precisely when language breaks down in the face of pain, when it becomes a mere skeleton of articulate speech, that feeling arises in Neoptolemus. He does not withdraw from the display of terrible pain and from the screams but rather feels a sudden affinity with Philoctetes: he sympathizes with him to the point of feeling Philoctetes' pain in his own body. In the following discussion, in which pain, language, sympathy, and hearing come together, I look back to my earlier considerations of Herder and Heidegger, and specifically the important connection between them. Philoctetes' wounded body as well as his damaged tongue converge with Neoptolemus' sympathy and his subsequent identification of and with Philoctetes' pain. The figure of Philoctetes, and specifically the pain-attack scene, stand at the center of this last chapter.

This scene (beginning from line 730 in Sophocles' play), includes two dire moments: first, we witness Philoctetes at the peak of his suffering, when pain overcomes him, wrecking his body before he falls to the ground, unconscious. Second, the scene presents the audience with the gradual disintegration of Philoctetes' language. Initially, Philoctetes speaks in recognizable words ("Child, it is killing me!"), but as his words fail him he utters increasingly incoherent exclamations and mere syllables such as "Ah, ah, ah!" and "APAPPAPA!" (in Meineck and Woodruf's translation) (*Sophocles, Philoc.* 730–820).

The Pain-Attack Scene

The pain-attack scene begins after Neoptolemus has promised Philoctetes he will rescue him from the island. Since however the young man is still completely loyal to his commander Odysseus, it is clear to the audience that he is lying to Philoctetes. But then something happens. Philoctetes suddenly suffers intense pain and freezes. Neoptolemus, surprised, repeatedly asks Philoctetes: "What is the matter?" Philoctetes replies: "Ah, ah, ah, ah!" and then "Ah! It goes through me, it goes through me!" then continuing with a series of exclamations: "A-a-a-a-a-h!" (*Sophocles, Philoc.* 730–750), in Meineck and Woodruff's translation: "ATATATA!" "APAPPAPA!" "PAPAPAPAP!" and in Storr's: "Ah me! ah me! ah me!"[5] This is a crucial moment as regards sympathy. Now Philoctetes' physical suffering constitutes a breach not only between himself and Neoptolemus but also between Philoctetes and his own language. Philoctetes' ability to express himself communicably collapses with this surge of pain. He is now completely cut off from Neoptolemus and is circumscribed by his pain and broken language. In Seamus Heaney's words, "There are no words for it. Only pity. Pity."[6]

In Sophocles' version, Philoctetes, afraid Neoptolemus too will leave him, seems to be intent on somehow reassuring the young man. He describes his pain as not too grave, for instance, and says he thinks it is better now (no worries, I'm fine, etc.). Very soon, however, these articulate sentences are interrupted by uncontrollable exclamations, "O gods!" and "Ah Ah Ah." There are some interesting interpretations of these cries of pain relating to the difficulties arising in the translation of the pain-attack scene, especially regarding Philoctetes' exclamations. According to Hall, Philoctetes' cries are in "extra-metrical" verse (rather than the usual Greek iambic-trimeter) so that his "Ah! Ah!" breaks the rhythmic flow of Philoctetes' earlier speech. Since it is "beyond words," Sophocles chooses these inarticulate sounds to express Philoctetes' pain, the common sounds produced by the bodies of both animals and human when they suffer.[7] Knox argues that the sustained rhythmic cry is untranslatable: there is no parallel way of representing these sounds of grief and cry in English. In Greek, such sounds are arranged into formal patterns expressing the height of suffering as well as the human endurance it calls for. The only way to render them into English, he writes, is by means of stage directions such as "a scream of agony, twelve syllables, three iambic metra long," and so forth.[8] Such an animal scream of pain, Knox writes, "is more than other human beings can stand; we live by forgetting that such pain exists, we shut it away in sound-proof rooms and dull it with drugs."[9] Philoctetes' cry, therefore, is not a matter of either direct bodily expression *or* linguistic expression: in it the two become inseparable.[10]

Hagi Kenaan considers this problem from a philosophical perspective in his discussion of what he calls the "personal" in language. Kenaan points out the abiding tendency of the philosophy of language (Anglo-American as well as continental) to establish the propositional form as the benchmark of our conception of language. This theoretical tendency has disconnected linguistic meaning from the relationship between an individual speaker and addressee, situating language solely in the correlation between a self-sufficient speaking subject and an object of reference. Language's content is therefore split from the particularity of the one who speaks: considering only the propositional dimension of language, this approach ignores the unique manner "in which you, being who you are, inhabit your speech." Language therefore remains disjoined from the particularity of our "tongue, breath, voice [and] body."[11] When Philoctetes cries out he does not express himself in propositional language and does not communicate, or capture his pain qua object of reference. These cries exactly allow his expression to sidestep the limitations of propositional language whose communicational qualities fail when it comes to expressing the personal, subjective presence of the individual.

In the case of the pain attack, it is precisely this alleged failure of proposition that allows Philoctetes to express his personal presence and Neoptolemus to respond to it. Let us look closely at Sophocles' pain-attack scene, taking into account the problem of sympathy.

NEOPTOLEMUS. Why are you silent like this, although nothing has been said, and stand as though struck dumb?

PHILOCTETES. Ah, ah, ah, ah!

NEOPTOLEMUS. What is the matter?

PHILOCTETES. Nothing grave. Come, my son!

NEOPTOLEMUS. Are you in pain because your sickness is with you?

PHILOCTETES. No, I think I am just getting better. O gods!

NEOPTOLEMUS. Why do you thus groan and call upon the gods?

PHILOCTETES. I am calling on them to come as preservers and be kind to us. Ah, ah, ah, ah!

NEOPTOLEMUS. What is the matter with you? Will you not tell me, but remain silent as you are? You seem to be in some trouble.

PHILOCTETES. I am lost, my son, I shall not be able to conceal my pain in your company. Ah! It goes through me, it goes through me! O misery, unhappy as I am! I am lost, my son! I am devoured, my son! A-a-a-a-a-h! I beg you, if you have a sword handy, strike at my heel! Lop it off quickly! Do not spare my life! Come, my son!

NEOPTOLEMUS. What is this sudden new thing that makes you cry out and groan so much?

PHILOCTETES. You know, my son.

NEOPTOLEMUS. What is it?

PHILOCTETES. You know, my boy!

NEOPTOLEMUS. What is the matter with you? I do not know.

PHILOCTETES. How can you not know? A-a-a-a-a-h!

NEOPTOLEMUS. The burden of the sickness is grievous!

PHILOCTETES. Grievous indeed, and indescribable! Come, take pity on me!

NEOPTOLEMUS. What shall I do?

PHILOCTETES. Do not take fright and betray me! It has come in person after a time, perhaps because it is weary of wandering, the sickness.

(*Sophocles, Philoc.* 730–759)

The scene begins when Neoptolemus notices that Philoctetes seems to have fallen silent. This silence, he says, is not in response to anything said to him and therefore part of a dialogue, but it marks instead a shut-down in the conversation. Rather than expressing, it disrupts expression. The initially close, friendly dialogue swiftly runs into a violent barrier where Philoctetes' speech fails,

Neoptolemus remaining baffled at his side. This unexpected change provokes a series of questions, all starting with the words "Why?" and "What?": What is this sudden new thing that makes you cry? Why do you groan? What is the matter with you? What shall I do? Neoptolemus evidently addresses the situation, trying to understand what has happened. But these questions, as if Neoptolemus is not taking in what is happening before his very eyes, manifest an insistence on his maintaining a safe distance from Philoctetes' pain, as if he is unable to see it.

Neoptolemus at this stage interprets the cries as articulate expression, seeming to understand them in the most literal way possible: when Philoctetes calls out "O gods!" it is an exclamation, not a statement, but Neoptolemus asks him why he calls for the gods. Philoctetes continues to cry (in different forms of "Ah ah"), but Neoptolemus ignores the cries and continues to ask him what is wrong, referring once again to Philoctetes' silence (*Sophocles, Philoc.* 730–761). There is, however, no silence at all. This is all the more peculiar since Philoctetes is not merely crying out; he turns to Neoptolemus directly, calling him "my son" and "my boy," as if the pain attack does not open a distance between the two men but creates an intimacy such as between father and son. Neoptolemus, however, remains unaffected, or perhaps even unaware of all this.

This inability to feel compassion for another, this deep insulation from another's cry of pain, brings to mind the epistemological incommensurability implied in what the Philosophy of Mind designates "the problem of other minds," whose exemplar is the feeling of pain. To recall, the problem at issue is the essential incongruity between our ability to know our own pains (immediate, irrefutable knowledge) and the knowledge we are capable of when other people's pains are concerned (mediated and doubtful). In the case of our pains, we have direct, irrefutable knowledge that is hardly distinguished from our bodily sensation; as for the pain of others, any attempt to ground knowledge immediately faces us with an epistemological impossibility. There is, therefore, a fundamental asymmetry with respect to knowledge, each having direct knowledge only of his own pains.[12]

When Neoptolemus asks Philoctetes what has happened to him, he is trying to understand, to know. The reiteration of these questions, however, points at his inability to know, at the epistemological gap between him and Philoctetes' suffering. Even if Philoctetes were to reply, Neoptolemus would not be able to know. Philoctetes, on the other hand, cannot share his pain by way of an explanation or proposition *about* his feeling; he can only feel it and immediately express it as he repeatedly utters the troubling sounds "Ah ah." Following the premises of the problem of other minds, the exchange in the pain-attack scene can be said to enact the essential impossibility for us to know or be certain about another's pain, thus confronting us with an essential hiatus between ourselves and others.[13] On the same lines, Neoptolemus' questions testify to the fact that he is shut out of Philoctetes' pain, that he cannot, in principle, have any *knowledge* of it. Neoptolemus continues to ask and Philoctetes' language continues to fail him. In other words, the cry of pain in this scene manifests most clearly and concretely what it means to argue that language "fails" in the face of intense pain, namely, that it stops functioning (functioning in this case meaning to communicate and impart information *about* pain). Pain reveals what a failed language sounds like.

Here I would like to argue that Sophocles' pain-attack scene presents a completely different picture. It is not concerned with the subject's distance from other people's pain and the skepticism it entails, but rather, with the deep sympathy and compassion arising precisely from the epistemological discrepancy between knowledge and feeling. Rebecca Comay points at the internal paradox of pain and its inarticulability when she writes that "the very thing that seems most to isolate us, to tear us away from the world, that can't and doesn't want to be shared, that seems to impede all connection and even to repel others with its relentless self-absorption and uncompromising drivenness—that is, pain itself—is the very basis of our most profound social bond. Suffering at once excludes and impinges on other people with its exorbitant ethical 'insistence.'"[14] Despite Neoptolemus' imperviousness, Philoctetes does not withdraw from this frustrating dialogue and insists on answering Neoptolemus' questions. This he does by repeating the phrases "You know" and "You must know" three times in the course of three lines (751–754). When Philoctetes says "You know," he does not mean that Neoptolemus can truly "know" his pain. Nobody can genuinely and fully "know" another's pain and Philoctetes is well aware of that. Yet he repeats the phrases "You know" and "How could you not know?" What is this knowledge that Philoctetes refers to here?

I consider this dialogue to exemplify the crucial connection between, on the one hand, the (im-)possibility to know another's pain (Neoptolemus does not understand, does not know), and on the other, the persisting demand that others know one's pain (Philoctetes' repeating "You know"). I would like to think about this connection through the perspective of Stanley Cavell's ideas about skepticism and acknowledgment.

Knowing and Acknowledging: Cavell

Cavell's discussion of acknowledgment stems from his long-standing interest in and interpretation of Wittgenstein's *Philosophical Investigations,* which he describes as the greatest philosophical work of the twentieth century. A famously central topic in the *Philosophical Investigations* is the problem of pain.[15] (Cavell even writes that pain is one of Wittgenstein's "obsessive examples.")[16]

Discussing the problem of criteria and their application (a problem standing in the background of Wittgenstein's critique of the referential structure of language), Wittgenstein introduces pain as his principal example, and justifiably so. Three problems intersect in the encounter of pain with language: the problem of criteria, the problem of certainty, and skepticism regarding other minds. In pain, these three fundamental epistemological issues present themselves with extreme pertinence: when confronting another person's pain, criteria never suffice to gain certainty (this is inherent to any encounter with pain as such). Pain is thus paradigmatic for a state in which the intrinsic gap between criteria and a validation of existence results in fundamental unknowability. However, this structure not only reveals the essential obstacles to our ability to "know" pain or validate its existence, but also and importantly, it illustrates our firm prejudice regarding the distinction between internal and external, private and communicable.[17]

Considering the question of how our words refer to our sensations, Wittgenstein maintains that the word "pain" does not describe our cry of pain (the inarticulate, immediate expression of pain) but replaces it.[18] Shifting the discussion from translation from one language to another, to movement between different forms of expression highlights another crucial point: it puts the categories of internal and external outside the discussion. The word "pain" no longer implies translation of an independent internal object into its external linguistic "name tag." According to Wittgenstein, such a configuration erroneously points at something "behind" the external expression, something that is allegedly the independent (and invisible) point of reference of this expression ("For how can I go so far," Wittgenstein writes, "as to try to use language to get between pain and its expression?").[19] Wittgenstein's alternative is thus to give up an internal object altogether and renounce what Cavell calls the "fantasy" of having access to any such object in the first place. Thus Wittgenstein avoids the misleading inner-outer binary and sets aside the illusion of our ability to "introspect" as if our internal states were subject to our observation, let alone the possibility to know other people's pains. This is not to say that Wittgenstein doubts the existence of pain or one's ability to feel it; the question of the certainty of inner states is not Wittgenstein's question at all. His focus is on the possibility to say something philosophically meaningful about such states. It is always helpful to remember that Wittgenstein's discussion is about language, expression, and meaning—and does not present ontological questions regarding the "objects" of language.[20]

Cavell's discussion of the problem of skepticism is far-reaching and has a whole range of implications for the history of philosophy generally as well as literature and tragedy in particular. In this discussion, pain plays a crucial role. This is partly because it is in the context of pain that the threat, even the danger, of skepticism becomes palpable. Nevertheless, Cavell's project is not to refute skepticism altogether but to convey the threat it poses to ordinary language philosophy. Skepticism enacts, in many ways, our drive to deny the conditions of human existence conceived of in terms of knowledge. For Cavell, understanding what it means to be human, to exist, is a constant attempt to face this fear of uncertainty and it therefore that for him the recognition of this fear is of the utmost importance, we could even say that it would be dangerous to deny it. "You might even take it as the mission of philosophy now to preserve rather than to turn aside the scandal of skepticism—as if this preservation is our access to the memory that we are, or meant to be, human, to live with stumbling."[21] Considered in light of Neoptolemus' position, which might be called skeptical, his misunderstanding and fundamental doubt of Philoctetes' pain is not merely an obstacle to overcome or a moral failure; it shows, rather, how pain reveals something important about our relationship with others.

In his "Knowing and Acknowledging," which is here my main reference point, Cavell analyzes the skeptical position according to which it is impossible for us to know another person's pain because of its internal, "private" nature, and this does not allow us to be certain that we have the same feeling, that we feel the pain *he* does.[22] The skeptic asks the right questions and points at the crux concerning pain as well as knowledge, but his conclusion is terrifying: it draws a clear and explicit boundary between what the other person feels and what we cannot feel with him, never able to feel the exact way that *he* does. When we understand these implications, "we are shocked," Cavell writes (*Acknow.* 246–247). We feel that we must refute the skeptic position. This is, however, a philosophical instinct that Cavell wants to pay closer attention to. His "In Quest of the Ordinary" provides an elaborate explanation. Skepticism, according to Cavell, triggers our drive to deny the conditions of human existence. Insofar as "that *denial* of the human is essential to what we think of *as* the human, skepticism cannot, or what I call the threat of skepticism must not, be denied."[23] This argument leads Cavell to understand philosophy's mission as that of preserving, rather than refuting, what he calls the scandal of skepticism. According to Cavell, the skeptic

> begins with a full appreciation of the decisively significant facts that I may be suffering when no one else is, and that no one (else) may know (or care?); and that others may be suffering and I not know, which is equally appalling. But then something happens, and instead of pursuing the significance of these facts, he is enmeshed—so it may seem—in questions of whether we can have the same suffering, one another's suffering. . . . He has, or seems to himself to have, discovered that unless we can share or swap feelings, we can't know what that person is experiencing (if anything). (*Acknow.* 247)

Cavell is not aiming here in the direction of eighteenth-century ideas such as Adam Smith's, according to which, since I cannot possibly know the other's pain as I am trapped within my own body, the only thing I have at my disposal is what Smith refers to as a sympathetic response, in its strict physical sense. Accordingly, though I am perhaps incapable of knowing, I can nevertheless with each and every fiber feel the other's pain in my own body. I can feel-for the other, by way of feeling the pain in myself.[24] Such a view would still border on the skeptic's position. Cavell offers an alternative. He does not ignore the problem which has, indeed, troubling implications; instead, he follows Wittgenstein's footsteps closely and offers an alternative that problematizes the epistemological point of view of the skeptic. Pain is not merely an inaccessible internal sensation that may be known with certainty or doubted. The problem of the pain of others is not an epistemological problem at all. Pain does not demand to be known; according to Cavell, it demands to be acknowledged.[25] With his introduction of acknowledgment into the scene of skepticism, Cavell can set aside the criteria of success or failure of communicative, referential language (which, following Wittgenstein, has no access to the internal or private) and move beyond the functions usually attributed to the utterance "I know." He suggests some other functions of "I know" relevant (or, not obviously irrelevant, as he puts it) in the case of knowledge of my own pain (e.g., knowing in the sense of being acquainted, confessing, or confirming) (*Acknow.* 255). These functions lead Cavell to establish "I know I'm in pain" as a statement that is not merely either certain or doubtful but rather an expression of exasperation that demands or calls for acknowledgment. In other words, the problem is not whether someone can know my pain, but whether he acknowledges *that* I am in pain.

In Cavell's sustained critique of skepticism, acknowledgment seems to provide his response to its dangers. However, when presenting the distinction between knowing and acknowledging, Cavell reminds us that acknowledgment is never an alternative to knowledge: it does not and cannot replace it. It is rather an interpretation of knowledge,[26] or, in Wittgenstein's words, "Knowledge is in the end based on acknowledgement."[27] In our case, acknowledging the pain of the other means comprehending the meaning of pain without reference to certainty, treating knowledge as having implications beyond certainty. Cavell's introduction of acknowledgment is therefore not a way to cope with an unanswerable question ("Is he *really* in pain?") but a suggestion, if not an imperative, to ask a wholly different question. At stake here is not certainty of the existence of pain but its meaning; and this meaning is never to be found independently in the endorsement of the physical event of pain as such. It always resides in the way in which pain emerges in the face of a response to it (be it from another human being, a community, or other less straightforward factors). Stephen Mulhall indicates that for Cavell, what the "grammar of pain" leaves out is not the pain itself vis-à-vis what Wittgenstein describes as the pain behavior but rather my response to this behavior: "The knowledge that such criteria confer imposes a call on me—for comfort, succor, healing; for a response which helps to assuage the pain or to acknowledge that it is unassuageable here and now."[28]

When, in the play, Philoctetes cries out inarticulately, it is clear that he does not explain his pain or communicate anything "about" it. I would even say that this is not his intention. Philoctetes' cry expresses exasperation, the very fact that he is in pain. In this sense, Neoptolemus' visit to the island changes nothing—no one can understand or know Philoctetes' pain and no one can relieve it. Yet something changes nevertheless. Neoptolemus may well be incapable of "knowing" Philoctetes' pain (the physical pain and the pain of abandonment); he may also not feel it, but he can acknowledge it. This is my reading of the words Philoctetes cries out at the height of his agony: "How can you not know?"

Cavell formulates a similar argument in his *Claim of Reason* in a wonderful passage concerning the fundamental problem with expressing our own pain and specifically the fear (rather than failure) it entails:

> My problem is no longer that my words can't get past his body to *him*. There is nothing for them to get to; they can't even reach as far as *my* body; they are stuck behind the tongue, or at the back of the mind. The signs are dead; merely working them out loud doesn't breathe life into them; even dogs can speak more effectively. Words have no carry. It is like trying to throw a feather; for some things, breath is better than strength; stronger. This is also something I meant by saying that voicing my criteria has to have the force of "call."[29]

Philoctetes realizes this. He knows Neoptolemus cannot have his own sensation, cannot feel it with the immediacy and intensity he does. But from the perspective of Cavell's thought, Philoctetes' fear and Neoptolemus' inability are not the end of the story. There is something unique about the experience of pain: on the one hand, the pain of another person seems to be similar to my own pains (at one time or another); on the other, Cavell claims (refuting Smith's position) that it is impossible for me to actually feel it, to make it my own. This internal paradox leads Cavell to argue that while the question of the incapacity to know another's pain is a real question, it has no answer. Simply stating that I cannot have the other's feeling is too weak for this predicament I experience and want to convey. We therefore need "to provide a characterization of this sense of incapacity *and* provide the reason for our insistence upon putting it into words" (*Acknow.* 262). I feel that we can know the same, that we share it, but "I am filled with this feeling—of our separateness, let us say—and I want you to have it too.

So I give voice to it. And then my powerlessness presents itself as ignorance—a metaphysical finitude as an intellectual lack" (*Acknow.* 263).

Das conveys this idea accurately when she argues that Cavell's interpretation of Wittgenstein unfetters us from thinking that our statements about pain (our own or another's) are to be evaluated in terms of certainty or doubt. The crux of Das' analysis here is that the "denial of the other's pain is not about the failings of the intellect but the failings of the spirit."[30] Something important comes up here: Cavell knows that since I cannot know, I will sometimes feel that I cannot acknowledge. Here is, however, one of the crucial, perhaps surprising, elements of his claim: acknowledgment means dealing with the pain of another—in other words, responding to it either by acknowledging it or by avoiding it. One way or another I have to be in touch with the other's pain. Acknowledgment is, in other words, something to be addressed, faced—even if it is not necessarily felt or actualized. Not responding is nothing less than perpetuating the violence generated by pain.

The relationship between Cavell's challenge of skepticism and Levinas' idea of the demand of suffering is of interest here, especially insofar as the connection between suffering and responsibility is concerned. Levinas describes the suffering of the other as a call or demand as well as an opportunity to suffer with the other, rather than a reason to withdraw or turn away from him. By foregrounding the response to the demand inherent to the other's suffering, Levinas grants it primacy over any epistemological compunctions.[31] He shows, moreover, that even a withdrawal from the other should not be understood as a mere opposite or negation of sympathy, but forms rather, a crucial indication of our primary moral responsibility toward the other, thereby emphasizing the ability of suffering to create a community based on mutual responsibility and commitment.[32]

At the peak of his pain attack Philoctetes passes out, and when he comes to his senses, Neoptolemus has undergone a change of heart. He tells Philoctetes the truth about Odysseus, and he confesses his own lies and their plan to steal his bow. But Philoctetes now grows suspicious. And here, an interesting reversal occurs. Trying to find out what has changed, it is now Philoctetes who keeps asking Neoptolemus questions like "Where has your talk strayed to?" and "What are you saying, my son? I do not understand" (*Sophocles, Philoc.* 896, 914). Philoctetes does not *know* what has changed or what Neoptolemus feels or thinks. He fears that Neoptolemus is disgusted by the wound and his screams and has changed his mind about rescuing him from the island (*Sophocles, Philoc.* 900–901). And indeed, Neoptolemus has changed his mind but in a completely different sense. He replies: "Everything is distasteful, when a man has abandoned his own nature and is doing what is unlike him!" and then "I shall be seen to be a traitor; that is what has long been paining me" (*Sophocles, Philoc.* 902–903, 906). Neoptolemus now embodies the moral change he had undergone.

It is now *he* who is disgusting and no longer the festering wound. His compassion for Philoctetes has revealed what he has kept hidden from himself: his choice to obey Odysseus at the expense of being cold-hearted toward another man who is—and this is important in the Greek context—similar to him in his aristocratic ancestry. Neoptolemus, unable to hide his inner turmoil any longer, cries out: "Ah!" (*Sophocles, Philoc.* 895). Like Philoctetes, he utters no articulate words but an exclamation.[33] Richard Eldridge's discussion of expressiveness in Cavell is important here. "Giving voice" to my pain, he writes, "implies not brute discharge alone, but further a making intelligible of how the human condition is present in one who has been moved to speak." To give voice is to achieve expressiveness, whose content and implications lie "beyond the communication of bits of information about the material world." In other words, it is not only acknowledgment that exceeds the mere knowledge or discursive understanding of another's pain but also, and importantly, the expressive act itself.[34]

Shifting the discussion of pain from knowledge to acknowledgment not merely opens up other possibilities for the one facing the other's pain. It also suggests something crucial about the sufferer himself. The sufferer does not expect us to come up with knowledge or some kind of confirmation of his pain (this would be senseless). He says: when I am in pain, I don't want you to know, I want you to acknowledge—not whether or not I am in pain, but the fact *that* I am in pain. More than enriching the way we think about the relationship between sufferer and the witness to suffering, Cavell's argument has important implications regarding the experience of pain itself. Suffering makes a claim on us, Cavell writes; "It is not enough that I *know* (am certain) that you suffer—I must do or reveal something (whatever can be done). In a word, I must *acknowledge* it, otherwise I do not know what "(your or his) being in pain" means. Is" (*Acknow.* 263). Cavell does not insist that we actually feel the pain of others, nor that we are filled with sympathy (or ought to be). Acknowledging is not about knowing, nor does it depend on whether or what we actually feel. It is, in other words, a moral stance.

The exchange between Philoctetes and Neoptolemus can therefore be read as not simply a failure of dialogue, of communicating one's pain, on the one hand, and of one's sympathy, in acknowledgment, on the other. Here Cavell's argument becomes pertinent:

> If one says that this is a *failure* to acknowledge another's suffering, surely this would not mean that we fail, in such cases, to *know* that he is suffering? It may or may not. The point, however, is that the concept of acknowledgment is evidenced equally by its failure as by its success. It is not a description of a given response but a category in terms of which a given response is evaluated. . . . A "failure to know" might just mean a

> piece of ignorance, an absence of something, a blank. A "failure to acknowledge" is the presence of something, a confusion, an indifference, a callousness, an exhaustion, a coldness. (*Acknow.* 263–264)

To recast this somewhat more elaborately than Sophocles and closer to Cavell's claim: it is impossible for you *not* to know because we are both human beings. And when a human being cries out in pain, you must understand his cry. You "know" my pain neither in the sense that you can enter my body and feel my infected foot nor because you once felt the same, but in the sense that you "know" what it "means" to be in pain—what it means to be human. Following Cavell, Neoptolemus might respond by saying, or feeling: "To know you are in pain is to acknowledge it, or to withhold the acknowledgment. I know your pain the way you do" (*Acknow.* 266). I do not want you, Neoptolemus, to know anything "about" my pain or validate it; I don't even expect you to help. I just want you to acknowledge the fact that here is a human being in agony, right next to you, and his agony makes a claim on you, on your humanity. I want you to acknowledge that we are both human beings and we are both vulnerable to pain: "I implore you, do not leave me here alone!" (*Sophocles, Philoc.* 808–809).[35]

Acknowledgment is so imperative precisely because it is not dependent on the moment of pain or the height of its expression. It is not a mere momentary response to a cry (physical or moral) but a complete transformation in our moral position. A momentary feeling of compassion that does not last is not what Cavell has in mind here. Moreover, acknowledgment is never conditioned: the event of pain and its expression do not condition the possibility of acknowledgment, nor does the presence of a specific person involved in a specific instance of pain. Neoptolemus awakens from his indifference not in the face of Philoctetes' initial cry of pain but when the fit of pain is over: it is only then that he expresses his acknowledgment. This is crucial. Mulhall provides a significant argument in this context: the implications of an *absence* of acknowledgment lie far beyond the specific event of pain, they touch on the grounds of our very existence: "If my pain is treated as unworthy of response by others . . . if my existence as a human being is denied in this way, then what does my existence as a human being amount to? In other words, if, through knowing others, I am implicated in their existence, then my existence is implicated in others' acknowledgements of me." My demand to be acknowledged amounts to nothing less than a demand to be human.[36]

For Cavell, acknowledgment is not about feeling (which he leaves behind together with knowledge) but concerns a practical commitment—not a sharing of pain, but an active response to it. The problem with skepticism is the distance it creates, whereas acknowledgment implies a decisive involvement, in this case, in Philoctetes' life. "What can I do?" Neoptolemus asks. "Don't leave me!,"

Philoctetes replies. Philoctetes' answer demonstrates precisely this: he does not seek the young boy's knowledge or feeling; he wants him to be there for him, to take part. Acknowledgment for Cavell goes beyond knowledge not because of a change in the hierarchy between them (it is not better or higher than knowing): it requires "that I *do* something or reveal something on the basis of that knowledge" (*Acknow.* 257).[37]

Gide's version especially reflects Cavell's understanding of acknowledgment. The encounter with Philoctetes, his figure as well as the story of his abandonment, leaves Neoptolemus stunned. Philoctetes' presence and words have taken root in his heart; he says, "While you were talking, I did not know what to answer, I listened, and my heart opened naively to your words. Ever since you stopped, I have kept on listening" (*Gide, Philoc.* 173). Throughout Gide's play, Neoptolemus repeatedly asks Philoctetes what virtue is; Philoctetes tries to explain but to no avail, until eventually he tells him: "Child! Ah, if I could only *show* you virtue." In the play's last scene we witness Neoptolemus trying to demonstrate to Philoctetes what virtue is: he tells him the truth and warns him against Ulysses; he hands him the sleeping potion Ulysses planned giving him. "Is this virtue?" asks Neoptolemus. "Is that what virtue is?" (*Gide, Philoc.* 174, 176). Philoctetes' reply manifests something of Cavell's insistence on defining acknowledgment not as a momentary feeling in the face of suffering but rather as an abiding moral stance: "Child! Superior virtue is attained only step by step; you are trying to make it at a leap" (*Gide, Philoc.* 176).

The play portrays the responsiveness of acknowledgment in several ways. The first is Neoptolemus' immediate response of touching Philoctetes. This moment marks Neoptolemus' acknowledgment: he realizes it, at first, by way of touch.[38] He is there, by Philoctetes' side, and reaches out to him. Even though Philoctetes refuses and rejects the possibility of touch (he hands Neoptolemus his bow instead), this is nevertheless a key moment as acknowledgment begins to arise in Neoptolemus. Another, more important actualization of Neoptolemus' commitment is his decision to replace his loyalty and obedience to Odysseus with an intimacy with Philoctetes. He confesses the lies and his own as well as Odysseus' scheme, testifying to his move to Philoctetes' side. This is what it means to be responsive to another's pain, to acknowledge it.

The Beauty of Language: Gide

As we have seen, Sophocles' pain-attack scene is a turning point in the play. It is when Philoctetes' words become violent, inarticulate noises, when his speech fails, that Neoptolemus is morally transformed. (This can be seen as the inverse of the events ten years earlier, when Philoctetes' wild cries of pain drove away his peers and soldiers, who ran rather than reaching out to him.) But this scene of extreme pain is not only crucial insofar as the problem of sympathy and compassion is concerned; it also forcefully manifests what it means for language, rather than to be demolished by pain, to be constituted by it, and for pain to be inextricable rather than categorically excluded from language.

We can, of course, account for Philoctetes' inarticulate cries by regarding them as instinctive and animal-like, depriving him of his communicative language and thereby, of his humanity. The moment appears to be one in which Philoctetes "loses" his language, when pain "overcomes" language and suppresses it. My argument is, however, different. Something irrefutably happens to Philoctetes' language but it would be inadequate to explain it away as some kind of failure to express or a mere lapse into a form of animal-being (as some analyses of this scene suggest). Although he does not use comprehensible words or full sentences here, Philoctetes *does* speak. His language does not refer to anything; it offers no propositional utterances or convey any type of semantic meaning. It speaks rather from the abyss of the expressionless, operating within the "strike" of language.[39] But this is, nevertheless, language.

My argument, touching on the question of sympathy as well as that of language, is grounded in André Gide's adaptation of the story: *Philoctetes; or, the Treatise on Three Ethics* (1898).[40] Gide's drama, whose original title was "Treatise of the Foul Wound (*Philoctète ou le Traité de l'immonde blessure*)" first appeared in the prestigious journal *Revue Blanche* in 1899. Although Gide did not intend the play for the stage, it was performed three times between 1919 and 1937. The play's subtitle refers to three ethical positions represented by its three protagonists, as Dugdale suggests: devotion to the other (Philoctetes), affection (Neoptolemus), and devotion to one's country (Ulysses). Gide's version is unique in his distinct depiction of Philoctetes. For Gide, Philoctetes is not simply trapped on the island for years, yearning to be rescued; or is he, as in Sophocles' version, a bitter, resentful man, wronged by the gods and his people and unable to forgive (even at the cost of his own life). Although Gide's Philoctetes is also abandoned and his pain is just as intense, his whole disposition is depicted differently. He is a calm, peaceful man, defined by his intimate kinship with the natural world. But most of all, Gide's *Philoctetes* tackles the question of language's relation to pain, foregrounding language's possibilities, rather than its impossibilities, as it faces the intensity and solipsism of pain.

As they wait for his arrival, Ulysses predicts to Neoptolemus what Philoctetes' response will be when he sees him. He will fly into a rage and curse, he tells Neoptolemus, blame me for abandoning him and wish for my death (*Gide, Philoc.* 167–168). Ulysses also predicts that Philoctetes will plead for his rescue. Ulysses is, however, completely wrong. When Philoctetes appears on stage and sees the two men, he is not resentful ("It is a great pleasure to see you again," he tells Ulysses); his lonely years on the island have engendered neither indignation nor a desire for deliverance—quite the opposite. After a long monologue in which he explains the beauty of his exilic life, Philoctetes declines Neoptolemus' and Ulysses' attempts to rescue him. He prefers his solitude, and after handing them his bow toward the end of the play, he realizes happily that his solitariness is permanent. This is conveyed first and foremost by means of the transformation in Philoctetes' language. Instead of describing his (inexpressible) pain or communicating it to others (no one is there, and even if there were, they could not have heard him)—Philoctetes' language now expresses a different form of pain, that of the natural world around him. Nature no longer functions as the "other" of human suffering, the empty, inhuman space in which the cry of pain can only echo itself. For Gide, nature itself suffers, its pain only revealing itself when Philoctetes himself cries it out (*Gide, Philoc.* 170). This alliance between language and nature is at the heart of Gide's Philoctetes who not only feels for nature as, to a certain extent, in Sophocles' version, but who prefers it to social life, which for him lacks any possibility of virtue (*Gide, Philoc.* 168–169). As Ulysses' ship sails away, Philoctetes stands calm and alone on a rock overlooking the sea and murmurs: "They will never come back; they have no more bows to seek. . . . I am happy" (178).[41] His voice, Gide describes in his stage directions, "has become extraordinarily mild and beautiful; around him flowers are showing through the snow, and birds from heaven come down to feed him" (*Gide, Philoc.* 178). Philoctetes' happiness depends on no one but himself and nature. The isolation that pain has enforced on him becomes a blissfulness.[42] Wilson associates Philoctetes' choice to remain on the island with his being a moralist, an artist, and a literary man, one "whose genius becomes purer and deeper in ratio to his isolation and outlawry . . . much relieved that there is no longer any reason for people to seek him out." Wilson ties this to his wider argument regarding the essential association between suffering and the gift of creativity, "the idea that genius and disease, like strength and mutilation, may be inextricably bound up together."[43]

But there is another important implication to Philoctetes' loneliness: it is closely and intimately related to his language. Recalling the terrible moment when he discovered he was abandoned on the island, Philoctetes recounts that while at first he cried and groaned, he soon discovered that there was no one there, "no ear to hear" his cries. So far, this description is largely similar to the one in Sophocles. But Gide's Philoctetes continues in an entirely different direction. In response to Ulysses' question of whether his loneliness caused him to fall silent over the years, Philoctetes replies "not at all":

> My suffering no longer needs words to make itself known, being known only to me. . . . Since I no longer use my complaint to manifest my

> suffering, it has become beautiful, so beautiful that it consoles me. . . . I express myself better now that I no longer talk with men. . . . I tried telling myself of my suffering, and if the sentence were beautiful, I was comforted accordingly. (*Gide, Philoc.* 169–170)

Philoctetes' enforced solitude and the eclipse of his communicative language have not impoverished him and turned him into an inarticulate animal; instead, it has functioned as a condition of possibility for a new linguistic expanse. Here, language is no longer constituted by and dependent on an intersubjective range of communication but rather materializes between Philoctetes and nature, in the nonhuman world around him. Philoctetes now experiences, and more importantly, can express not his own pain but the pain of nature. "Nature seemed the image of my distress; it seemed that I was nature's voice and that the mute rocks were waiting for my voice to tell their illnesses," he tells Ulysses; "I gradually got the habit of crying out the distress of things, rather than my own" (*Gide, Philoc.* 170).

These two forms of pain, the human and the natural, thus unite not on the plane of sensation but on that of *expression*. Gide thereby challenges one of the most established assumptions about pain and its expression: When someone succeeds or fails in expressing pain, it is always his or her *own pain* that is in question. Gide's Philoctetes demonstrates a wholly different structure: while he may fail in articulating his own pain, this failure becomes the condition of possibility for expressing another's pain (in this case, the pain of nature, an expressive possibility not limited to the human realm). In terms of the earlier mentioned problem of other minds, the pain of the other beyond merely being known or doubted, or even acknowledged, can also be expressed. Such expression is, in fact, a form of sympathy, an expressive sympathy, just as in the resounding echo in Herder's account of joint human and natural linguistic expression.

Gide's poetic Philoctetes, and Sophocles' account of the pain-attack scene are deeply consonant. Both poignantly present the failure of language, and in both, the failure does not amount to the destruction of language or humanity; rather, it is the opposite. In Sophocles, failure occurs where Neoptolemus' sympathy surges up at the end of the pain-attack scene—that is, precisely when Philoctetes' language fails. Indeed, as I show, it is only when Philoctetes' articulate phrases turn into howls ("Ah! Ah!") that sympathy emerges. Gide's account takes this further when, excluded from the human realm of communication, no longer able to say anything *about* pain, Philoctetes does not respond by withdrawing into a silent solipsism; rather, it is exactly then that he forms his unique expressive intimacy with the natural world.

This intimacy or kinship is made possible by two important features: first, nature, like him, suffers pain and is inexpressive; and second, Philoctetes' ability to respond to nature by way of expressing its pain is conditioned by his own pain, his suffering being. Moreover, the crux of the kinship between man and nature here is language: in Sophocles, the collapse into expressive inarticulate utterances; in Gide, a reopening of language that becomes beautiful in its very noncommunicativeness. Another point to think of here is the interesting reversal between Sophocles and Gide: in the first, language's failure in the face of pain (Philoctetes) gives birth to sympathy (Neoptolemus); in the second, language's failure to communicate is the origin of a language whose beauty inheres in that it no longer expresses one's own pain (Philoctetes) but the pain of others (Nature).

Gide and Cavell share another association constituted by the question of the collapse of language and the problem of sympathy. They approach the relationship between pain, language, and sympathy differently. Cavell's argument is unequivocally intersubjective. It challenges the epistemic framework dominating the problem of other minds, namely, the idea that there is an inherent gap between the expression of our own pain and the possibility of others to know it with certitude and let go of any intuitive doubts. Instead, Cavell suggests that although our pains cannot be known by others nor their certainty established, they nevertheless lay a claim, pose a demand. When we cry out in pain we do not demand knowledge or belief from others but rather their acknowledgment. This, for Cavell, occurs in the intermediate space between two persons: one expressing, the other acknowledging.

Gide's case is more complex. In his account, it is precisely Philoctetes' deprivation of a human sphere from which he can demand and receive sympathy that opens up a wholly new realm of connections, namely, between Philoctetes and everything on the island that is not human. Removed from any social domain, Philoctetes now knows the pain of nature that is deprived of language, and he expresses what was never itself endowed with a possibility of expression. Gide does describe a sphere marked by sympathy and, specifically, expression (Philoctetes expresses pain as well as sympathy); but it is a sympathy situated outside the human realm. Philoctetes' own unanswerable suffering gives him access to nature's pain and enables him to express it, yet this facility is made possible by the barrier put on his own human expression.

Gide's version, however, is not limited to the question of human versus inhuman sympathy but is closely related to Gide's conception of language in the face of pain and isolation. When we bring Gide's Philoctetes together with Elaine Scarry's work (which I discussed in detail in the previous chapters), an important distinction emerges. According to Scarry, physical pain destroys language and hence the possibility of maintaining a relationship with the world (this is what is meant by her book's subtitle "*The Making and Unmaking of the World*"). For Gide, pain may penetrate and undeniably color our experiences; but rather than causing language's destruction, pain reveals something about its conditions of possibility. Language is, no doubt, undermined by pain, and violently so. However, this violence has surprising implications. Pain is double-faced: it violates language but at the same time allows it to cure itself by way of reflecting upon itself.[44] Language, at this point, no longer depends on external anchors (referring to this or that object of reference) but can express itself alone.

Philoctetes' isolated existence on the island has not dried up his language: it has not reached its limit or receded in utter impotence: "I express myself better now that I no longer talk with men," he tells Ulysses (*Gide, Philoc.* 170). On the contrary, from the very collapse and failure to propositionalize, Gide's Philoctetes has rediscovered language: "I learned that words are more beautiful when they ask for nothing. With neither ears nor mouths around me, I used only the beauty of my words" (*Gide, Philoc.* 170). The beauty Philoctetes describes here is a beauty that is possible only when language does not "function," cannot communicate, when it isn't conditioned by being heard or responded to: when it "asks for nothing." His utterances, Philoctetes explains, cannot be repeated (they are not made of words) or propagated. It is only then that he understands that the "intimate flame" that animated his speech (for it was "merely" communicative and referential, dependent on what was external to it rather than on itself) is now slowly shrinking. Philoctetes' language of pain has its own independent, inner flame, its own inner force (*Gide, Philoc.* 171). Instead of actualizing possibilities (of communication), it has become its own condition of possibility. Language becomes autonomous when it encounters pain, because pain is no longer its object of reference. In that sense, language "learns" something from pain, from its solipsistic and staggering nature, from the power of its self-centered essence, which cannot and does not want to depend on anything but itself.[45]

"Language, Indeed Every Language, Is the Language of Pain"

I am indebted here to Werner Hamacher whose work is closely related to my own thoughts about the relationship between language and pain.[46] Hamacher has contemplated pain throughout his work, more or less explicitly. But it is neither in the physical nor mental sense that pain interests him. For Hamacher, pain and language are uniquely interconnected: "Language," he writes, "indeed every language, is the language of pain."[47] The roots of this peculiar claim can be found in another of Hamacher's "95 Theses on Philology."[48] In thesis 52 he quotes the following lines from Celan's "Tübingen, January": "he could, | if he spoke of this | time, he | could | only babble and babble | over, over | againagain. | | ('Pallaksh. Pallaksh.') [nur lallen und lallen,/immer-, immer-/zuzu ('Pallaksch. Pallaksch.')]" (*Theses* 34). Philology, according to Hamacher, would respond to these lines by refusing any attempts "at measurement through a norm of language that shatters in them" (*Theses* 34). The babble, the stammer, are not pathological in any way; rather, they voice a disorder that belongs to language as such, a language of pain which does not, in Hamacher's words, "bring pain to language but language to pain" (*Theses* 34).

In 2014, Hamacher wrote me a letter in which he rejected the view that treats language as a way of expressing an internal feeling—for instance, the pain felt when a friend departs. Let me quote a few lines from this letter:

> I do not think of language in terms of expression. [I reject] the interpretation of language as a way of expressing something like feelings, emotions etc. The notion of expression relies on a limit between inside and outside, one might call it a "spatial metaphor," but the placement and the very possibility of drawing such a limit is entirely dependent on language: language draws the line between in and outside, and therefore language itself cannot be subjected to this partition. It is the partitioning, the imparting, the spacing. Human space is lined up and out-lined by language, and so is time. In a kind of reverse action, language may become subjected to what it has done, subjected, that is, to the space it has opened and the time it has given. Then, and only then, it can appear as "expressing" something.[49]

The problem with expression lies, according to Hamacher, in the assumption that language is positioned on the border between inside and outside—walling off the hiddenness of internal emotions and feelings from the outspokenness of words. Language, however, does not surrender to this separation but constitutes it. Put differently, language, rather than being expressive, emerges as the condition of the possibility of expression. Distancing us from communicative speech, Hamacher's understanding of language leads the way into the space of interruption, of the strike of, and in, language: of the partition it constitutes rather than surrenders to. Instead of actualizing its propositional possibilities, language becomes its own condition of possibility, speaking only itself. These arguments bring Hamacher's thought into a special intimacy with the experience of pain whose intensity renders it impervious to objectification and therefore cannot be represented or communicated. It is content-less and can thus express only itself. In that sense, language "learns" something from pain, from its solipsistic and staggering nature, which does not and cannot be dependent on anything but itself.

It is helpful to take a glance at the opening of "The Second Inversion," where Hamacher criticizes conceptions of language represented by Aristotle, in which linguistic utterances perform mainly as propositions directly referring to independent objects or states of affairs. What troubles Hamacher is that according to such "unreflective" views, language is "explained away as an empty gesture" at the moment of its encounter with "the power of the factual."[50] Language is thus destined to disappear when things themselves become present. Understood as a shadow of reality, language is therefore an apparatus doomed to be trapped in the continuous movement of mere empty repetition and representation, of that which is posited vis-à-vis language. Language can thus only produce statements *about* something else, about that which is defined as not being language's own.

Hamacher's work is a constant, persistent movement against such linguistic conceptions.[51] His alternative is pronounced most forcefully in his work on Paul Celan. From within his readings of Celan's poems as well as the poet's famous "Meridian" speech, Hamacher traces and delineates an understanding of language that provides an alternative to the tradition rooted in Aristotle. Language, no longer defined on the basis of its semantic or propositional functions, can express itself to the fullest precisely in the absence of such functions. Its essence is therefore manifested in a "chronic retreat" from language's referential and semantic functions, when it is freed from its persistent dependence on the factual.

It is in Celan's poetry that Hamacher finds an expression of language as such, in itself, autonomous and independent from anything external to it, be it an object, addressee, or state of affairs that language expresses in a proposition. The essence of language is therefore revealed precisely in its withdrawal from the world of its objects of reference, "just as the functions of the sign break down in the face of an 'object' such as an abyss, death, or nothingness, conventional units of meaning—words and sentences, strophes, which are also turns—likewise dissolve, having been infected, as it were, with this death, and they thus leave room for an altered form of speaking and for the interruption of speaking itself."[52] In other words, the strength of poetic language is exposed and expressed when such language faces its own inability to function as the representational "shadow" of an object, when it encounters what is devoid of any form of objective presence. In these sites where propositional language can only negate ("dead" is "not alive," etc.), poetic language possesses the force to withstand the abyssal without being silenced or merely negated. This is when Celan's poetry asserts language's conditions of possibility only as the conditions that make the stability of its semantic subsistence and referential functions impossible. But how can it represent such absence? According to Hamacher, poetic language can do so when the expanse of language's functions is broadened: when language is no longer a mere instrument of representation but instead is expressive of its own conditions; it no longer eloquently speaks but begins to stammer. Its stammering, its internal interruption, is now completely independent, referring only to itself. Language faces language—and its autonomy is forcefully established.

Hamacher's renowned "Afformative, Strike" is pertinent in this context. In his interpretation of Walter Benjamin's 1921 "Critique of Violence (Zur Kritik der Gewalt)," Hamacher introduces what he calls the "afformative."[53] According to Hamacher, language is not a medium that can be measured against an objective state of affairs, "a standard verifiable independently of this medium and already available outside itself" (*AF* 1144). Language articulates, rather, the mediacy that precedes the possibility of distinguishing "true" from "false" and therefore cannot be subject to this distinction which it itself constitutes (*AF* 1143). Following Benjamin's criticism of the "bourgeois" or instrumental conception of language, Hamacher develops Benjamin's suggestion of an immediate, pure language. Such a conception of the linguistic would reject any form of communication or proposition, offering instead an emphasis on language's "affirmative" aspect rather than its performative dimensions. The afformative therefore is the pre-performative and pre-propositional (*AF* 1143–1144, 1139, n.12).

But although the afformative is not a simple linguistic act, it is never, Hamacher emphasizes, simply banished from the sphere of acts or deprived of any relation to that sphere. "The afformative," Hamacher sums up, "is the ellipsis which silently accompanies any act and which may silently interrupt any speech act" (*AF* 1139, n.12). Always a condition but never an actualization, it is the "pre-" of language, the abstention from action. The essence of language is, accordingly, not limited to its representational, semantic, and referential functions. Nor is it found in its ability to "perform," that is, to constitute the real rather than merely to describe it. And therein lies yet another important difference between Hamacher's conception and Aristotle's. For the latter, language is ironically revealed when it succeeds in evaporating in the fact of its objects of reference; in Hamacher's case, language has to fail in this function so that it can emerge in all its grandeur. It has to fail in order to appear. In other words: instead of succeeding in order to disappear, it has to fail so that it can materialize in its purity.

This takes us back to Hamacher's aforementioned letter: language does not surrender to the partition between internal and external; it constitutes that partition in the first place. The vehement encounter between language and pain is not about language expressing or not being able to express pain as some internal content, hidden behind the barrier of the body or our doubtful relation to "other minds." It is the partition itself that is at stake here, constituted and manifested. Pain, therefore, does not mark the failure or collapse of language; rather, it allows a manifestation of the strength of language, its boundlessness: it brings forth its possibilities, the very conditions that allow it to be language. In pain, to use Hamacher's categories," language does not speak"; it cannot produce a proposition corresponding to a factual state of pain. Language is also incapable of "performing" in the face of intense pain and can barely "touch" it with its weak words and sentences. But, following Hamacher, we cannot speak here of a "performative contradiction," since such contradictions can arise only from within a linguistic system that has already been established as instrumental, as measured by its effectiveness.[54] The appearance of language is marked by its own failure.

In "Other Pains" (*Andere Schmerzen*)," a text Hamacher never finished and which was published posthumously, we find important remarks about the relationship between pain and the strike of, and in, language (*Pains* 963–989). Along with Pindar, Cicero, Seneca, Kant, Hegel, and Valéry, he devotes a short subchapter to Sophocles, and more specifically to his *Philoctetes*. Hamacher is not preoccupied with the hero's unjust suffering or with questions of sympathy and acknowledgment. He is entirely absorbed in the way in which Philoctetes' pain does not, and cannot, function as an internal object to which extraneous language is intentionally directed. In this text Hamacher considers the unique structure of pain and suffering, which becomes, as the text develops, the structure of language as it encounters pain. Both language and pain are shattered by their own excessiveness. The experience of pain, according to Hamacher, indicates what is measureless throughout the time it is endured, pain having "a measure all its own and thus no measure at all; a pain that can be compared with no other and therefore remains immeasurable" (*Pains* 967). This is why suffering is solitary: since its magnitude is incommensurable with anything but itself, it belongs to the sufferer alone and fails to allow any relationship with others. It cannot be open to their sympathy or the possibility of a community. Pain here *constitutes*, rather than being *constituted as*, the object of language. Philoctetes is "sick with sickness" and "suffers suffering": formulations that reflect *nosei noson*, a "cognate accusative," an intransitive grammatical structure that achieves emphasis through repetition (*Pains* 967). For Hamacher, Philoctetes does not suffer a single terrible, pain among all possible pains: he suffers from suffering itself (*Pains* 967). Similar to the structure of *nosei noson*, in which there is no object, no independent content and only a repetition of the nominative, here too, Philoctetes is "thoroughly affected by being affected, struck by being struck, passive before being passive. He experiences, in short, experience" (*Pains* 968).

Considering the relationship between pain and the possibility of experience, Hamacher argues that the Kantian conception of knowledge is conditioned by the subject's capacity to posit, a capacity that eludes the sufferer, who has lost his ability to hold the world together, as posited, thus not experiencing himself as a constituting subject (in the Kantian sense) but experiences an occurrence preceding every object, yet also every subject of experience" (*Pains* 969). Although pain is experienced, it is not *part* of experience. Put in terms of "Afformative, Strike," pain is "pre-subjective, pre-objective, and thus prepropositional, the occurrence of mere suffering is pre-spatial, pre-temporal, pre-worldly" (*AF* 1135). Gide's Philoctetes speaks language itself, and therein lies its beauty. Hamacher's Philoctetes experiences his mere experience. In both cases, *what* he experiences, Hamacher writes, is "indistinguishable from experience itself" (*Pains* 968). And here, Hamacher's description of the suffering of Philoctetes is remarkably close to Gide's account of his Philoctetes' language that encompasses no content and finds no support in its propositional functions (*Pains* 968).

"Pallaksh.Pallaksh" is, accordingly, a "memorandum of a language that would be human in a different way—a language of pain which can only say that it is allowed to babble but which injures its own law: which does not bring pain to language but language to pain" (*Theses* 34). Language brought to pain means that language cannot express pain as its object, because in the state of intense pain the gap between language and its objects no longer exists. Language now faces pain as what is internal to it, inseparable from it. It is not a language *about* pain; it is nothing other than pain itself. "Language, indeed every language," Hamacher writes," is the language of pain" (*Pains* 965).

6

Language Pangs

A Third Paradigm

Herder's *Treatise* and *Critical Forests*, Heidegger's *On the Essence of Language*, as well as Philoctetes' story in its many versions, all the way to Gide's *Philoctetes* and finally, Cavell—are all milestones in this book's long stretch. At this point we must glance back at the two paradigmatic views on the relationship between pain and language that have come to dominate how we think about their intersection. The crux of the first paradigm is the destructive nature of pain, and it emphasizes the violence pain inflicts on body, psyche, and sense of self. The second paradigm has to do with the unique manner in which pain isolates us from others, creating an abyss between those in pain and those witnessing it. Pain destroys, therefore, not only our bodies but also the possibility of our relationship with others.[1]

Thinking the two paradigms together we could say that by destroying us, in all respects, pain also destroys our ability to communicate and share it. Inasmuch as pain becomes inseparable from us, it imposes an absolute separation from others. However, these two paradigms not only concern the experience of pain (its consequent destruction and isolation) but also the importance of their relation to language. Pain is the experience with perhaps the most powerful connection to language and expression, making it always and essentially an experience of language: first, by virtue of the collapse of articulate language in the face of pain; second, through the strong connection between the experience of pain and the urge to express it, on the one hand, and the consummate impossibility of saying anything about pain, describing it, or communicating it, on the other. Pain therefore demands expression while preventing its articulation. But in these paradigmatic views, both, beyond everything, construe the relationship between pain and language as antagonistic, a violent confrontation, either-or, all-encompassing, or destructive. This fierce antagonism, however, reveals that pain is most accurately defined in relation to language, and language makes itself manifest in relation to the experience of pain. In other words, it is exactly because their point of departure is in violent opposition that the association between language and pain is undisputable.

The hold of these two paradigms was gradually attenuated in the course of the chapters discussing Herder, Rousseau, Heidegger, Sophocles, Cavell, and Gide. None of these writers refutes the violence pain does to language and our relations with others, to our bodies and psyches, but none of them considers this the end of the story: on the contrary, this violence rather constitutes its beginning. What the two paradigms treat as the ruins of language, its discordant fragments or debris, this line of thinkers reveals to be the exact opposite: this irreducible antagonism and incongruity guarantees the strength and abundance of language and the living force of expression. In addition, rather than isolating us from others, defeating the possibility of sympathy, pain's violence constitutes it, deepening our bond with others, which now no longer depends on the success or failure of our communicative abilities. Philoctetes' story stands out not only by exemplifying alternative conceptions of pain and language but most of all, by showing that the relationship between them is not one-sided and exhausted by a strict, unidirectional interaction. Instead, it opens up an extensive, varied range of expression.

The philosophy of language in the twentieth century has taught us to consider language from two main perspectives. The first, in a long tradition beginning with Aristotle, conceives of language as having a fundamentally propositional structure, its utterances referring to objects or states of affairs, their role limited to their semantic and referential functions that are forever dependent on the objects they stand for or seek to represent.[2] Following up on my discussion of Hamacher in chapter 5, such a conception renders language dispensable as it encounters its objects. Language can thus only produce statements *about* something else, about that which is defined as not being language's own. According to Hamacher, such semantics-based linguistic theories can only propound an aporetic verdict: "Language does not speak; it has nothing to say, only itself or its disappearance."[3]

The second dominant conception of language is famously represented in the work of J. L. Austin who offers an alternative to this merely representational and propositional conception of language.[4] Austin's linguistic theory of the performative utterance criticizes and challenges the philosophical bias that has fostered a limited understanding of language on the basis of its referential, semantic structure. Austin suggests that we rethink the boundaries of language so that they encompass not only what language describes or refers to in reality but also what it can *do*. Instead of stating a proposition about something that exists, language does something additional with its words; it makes something happen (saying "I do" during a marriage ceremony is one of Austin's famous examples). That is, in order for us to determine whether a linguistic action or performance is successful (Am I now married or not?), we measure with reference to reality and never in solely linguistic terms.[5] In the context of Austin's performative and the interesting philosophical debate around it (most prominently, the contributions by John Searle and Jacques Derrida), Hagi Kenaan criticizes the philosophy of language (Anglo-American as well as continental) for its comprehensive focus on success and neglect of failure which has led to a misleading tendency to equate a "successful" utterance with the achievement of communication.[6]

Considering these two philosophical arguments about language—the propositional and performative—we arrive at a similar problematic. Although Austin's performative utterances pose a substantive challenge to the referential and propositional conception of language, his theory nevertheless crucially assumes language's intrinsic dependence on external reality. The performative does not describe the factual or objective reality but rather creates it; its criteria, however, still involve the connection between linguistic utterance and an objective, external state of affairs. While language may be exempt from the requirement to represent the factual, it remains entangled with it through the performative utterance's characteristic quality of transforming actual reality. In this sense, these two dissonant theories—referential versus performative approaches to language—share some substantial presuppositions grounded in the perceived interdependence between language and states of affairs: in terms of the first conception, language describes states of affairs; in terms of the second, it creates them.[7]

The paradigms that construe pain's encounter with language as being overwhelmingly destructive and isolating are both grounded, strongly but also blindly, on criteria of success or failure. From such a perspective, pain cannot be described, referred to, or fully communicated; language, whether propositional or performative, does not furnish a way out of pain; it cannot relieve or alter it. In this sense language cannot perform in the face of intense pain, presenting us with a linguistic abyss. The abyss, however, is not only limited to speech and its relation to pain as its object of reference. It goes deeper and cuts off from others those in pain struggling to communicate their suffering, leaving the others unable to respond—a failure of proposition as well as communication. It should be noted that both these domains in which failure takes place—the propositional as well as the communicative—hinge on the premise that language is intrinsically tied up with an external world: objects of reference as well as addressees. My main argument in this book challenges such views and comes to argue instead that the relationship between language and pain is not exhausted by these functions and demands a different outlook.

In Conclusion

It is here that I would like to bring Herder's *Treatise* back into the discussion. As I have shown in detail throughout the book, Herder's reference to Philoctetes is misleadingly marginal. Although this figure seems to disappear after a few pages, Philoctetes functions as far more than a mere illustration for Herder, and his presence can be felt on every page of the *Treatise*. In the span between the book's first and last chapter—between the allusion to Philoctetes and the detailed elucidation of the figure and his story—the book's central arguments, and specifically those pertaining to the relationship between the experience of pain and linguistic expression, are elaborated.

To begin at the very beginning: Herder understands the origin of language as a purely somatic moment. Using pain as his primary paradigm, he presents the primordial, immediate cries of pain as inseparable from the sensation they express. Pain, therefore, is not language's object of reference nor does it amount to a particular, given state of affairs that language attempts to capture and describe. The cry of pain, furthermore, does not function as a propositional utterance and in no way endeavors to communicate any content *about* pain. In this manner, the body, rather than being what language has to overcome in order to come into being, becomes the very site of its origin. Language is not independent from sensation, pointing at it; instead, the body becomes the axis on which two forms of expression intersect: linguistic expression and the expression of pain.

But Herder's treatise on the origin of language makes another, even more significant claim. Although he explicitly separates between the two languages under discussion—the primordial language of sensations and reflective human language—Herder's claim regarding this partition is misleading. As I have shown in detail, a conception of language as not being essentially communicative, but rather expressive, is manifest not only in the immediate cry of pain but also stands at the heart of Herder's description of human language. In other words, the *Treatise* demonstrates that the expression of pain is not antecedent to human language and is not to be conceived of as a pre-language or primitive stage in any way. "These groans, these sounds," Herder writes, "are language" (*Treatise* 66/*AS* 697). The implications are radical: immediate, instinctive cries are themselves language, and moreover, they are not left behind when human language enters the scene. Human language is not defined as an overcoming of instinctive animal cries but is interrelated with them insofar as both are expressive rather than being referential or communicative.

Considering the story of Philoctetes in this frame of reference suggests, I argue, a unique, perhaps surprising, reading of the pain-attack scene. The sudden collapse of articulate linguistic utterance into a series of vehement, savage exclamations does not imply that Philoctetes' pain has deprived him of his language and, thereby, his humanity. It does not turn him into a speechless animal and, most important, does not confine him to an enclosed, solipsistic realm of pain that denies entry to others. If the question of humanity nevertheless arises in the context of Philoctetes' cries of pain, rather than being pertinent to his own person, it implicates his soldiers and fellow commanders who abandoned him not only *when* he was in extreme pain but *because* of his pain and its expression, in direct response to his unbearable screams. For Herder, a crying man is not characterized by his animality, nor is the articulate, speaking man necessarily distinguished by his humanity.

Philoctetes also bears out something else in Herder's argument regarding the relationship between the two languages. In the *Treatise* Herder admits that although the human shares the original language of sensations with the animal, this kinship has come to be subdued in reflective human language. And yet there are distinct moments in which the language of sensations, the "mother-tongue" (*mütterlichen Sprache*), resounds with all its vigor and "reassumes its right." This occurs, according to Herder, in moments of extreme sensation and feeling, such as revenge, fright, joy, and pain (*Treatise* 67/*AS* 699). Philoctetes makes contact with the origin of language when pain strikes him. The immediate language of pain cannot be simply contemplated or theoretically considered: its presence, or reemergence, is dependent on these extreme moments to which we are sometimes (rarely, according to Herder) subjected. It is then that our mother tongue expresses itself rather than as a result of our volition to voice it. Thus, Philoctetes is conjured in the *Treatise* not as the embodiment of a man-animal but as a man whose intense pain causes him to touch, physically, the original moment of language. Pain is therefore not the end or demise of humanity and language; rather, it indicates their common origin.

This structure has the potential of raising some critical reservations as it is difficult to defend the argument that an immediate, physical cry of pain qualifies as linguistic articulation. To clarify this difficulty, I do not understand Herder here as simply extending the sphere of language so that, with a somewhat postmodern gesture, everything becomes language, nothing escapes language, and the like. An alternative understanding of Herder's claim can be found, away from his account of the original language of sensations, in his description of reflective human language. Herder constitutes reflective language not by way of speech or communication but through its nature as an expressive apparatus, in which not only the cry remains central but also a person's ability to *hear* it. By foregrounding the production and hearing of sounds, Herder poses a rigorous challenge to the customary configuration in which language is positioned in an intersubjective plane with the inherent separateness between human beings demanding that they "invent" language as a means of straddling the communicative divide. Insofar as the cry of pain is inseparable from language, it cannot become its object of reference; consequently, it remains outside any propositional and communicative apparatus. It does, however, constitute a very strong form of interrelatedness, which is neither semantic nor communicative in kind. This crucially hinges on Herder's emphasis on the role of hearing, rather than speech, in language.

Contrary to the first paradigmatic conception, the immediate cry of pain does not exclude us from the social, communicative sphere, condemning us to perpetual isolation. Although Herder does not think of the cry as imparting information or any other articulate content, neither does he regard language as ruining the very possibility of relationship to anything or anyone external to pain. In this sense, his theory of language cannot be further away from the core issue of the problem of other minds: our inability to propositionally refer to pain or describe it should not suggest that those not in pain are excluded from the one suffering it, even from the very sensation of pain involved. For Herder, the original immediacy of language belongs with the cry of pain but pertains no less to the immediate response it elicits. When someone cries out in pain, the question of doubt immediately emerges: for those suffering, pain cannot be doubted; for those unaffected by it, pain is nothing but doubtful. This is where Herder's theory of sympathy stands out. The possibility, or for that matter, impossibility, of sympathy is uprooted from questions of certainty, doubt, or our communicative skills. For Herder, the cry of pain induces an immediate natural response: any cry of pain is essentially interrelated with a resonance or response—both firmly situated in the acoustic domain. Herder relies on a musical metaphor, comparing the sympathetic relationship to that of two reverberating strings. His conception of the whole of nature's participation in pain allows us to abandon the hypothesis that pain belongs merely to the body suffering it. Under the rule of sympathy, a single pain is a communal one.

It is clear how this connects to the figure of Neoptolemus. His transformation at the end of the pain-attack scene can be interpreted to signal a paradigm shift: instead of regarding Philoctetes' exclamations as evidence of the destruction of articulate language, leading in turn to a rift between the two men, the transition from words to cries should be read as the critical moment of rapprochement. Neoptolemus' insistent, concerned questions about the sudden change in Philoctetes derive from the perspective of strictly propositional, communicative language: Neoptolemus wants to *understand*. This radically changes at the end of the scene, when Philoctetes falls to the ground unconscious. Now Neoptolemus realizes that his questions cannot be posed in an epistemic framework, namely, that the problem at stake is not whether he has sufficient information to know what has happened. He needs to understand, but differently. The discord between the question (What happened?) and the answer (Ah ah ah ah) is the outcome of the fact that they exist in entirely different realms. And with this realization he sees that he, in fact, *does* know Philoctetes' pain, that he does *understand*. This understanding is not epistemic or communicative or propositional; it is rooted in the nature of sympathy: the point here is not knowledge but acknowledgment. Pain, in other words, does not impede sympathy but constitutes it. Put differently, sympathy not only does not clash with the inarticulate cry of pain; it depends on it.

Here Cavell's notion of "acknowledgment" is pertinent: the problem of the relationship between pain and language is not epistemic (i.e., to be considered in terms of the problem of other minds); it is a problem of sympathy. It has to do with our ability to feel, not with what we are able or unable to know. Acknowledgment, he writes, is not a response that emerges in the context of the attempt to know; it is not mutually exclusive with knowledge. To this Cavell writes that failing to know can be described as an absence, a blank, whereas a failure to acknowledge implies "the presence of something, a confusion, an indifference, a callousness, an exhaustion, a coldness" (*Acknow.* 264). Neoptolemus' transformation does not have to do with identifying with Philoctetes or with overcoming the breach between them and sharing his pain. Neoptolemus responds. Instead of emotional indifference and a rigidly insistent demand to know the other's pain, Neoptolemus acknowledges that Philoctetes is in pain and thereby also that he is committed to him (not his pain). The importance of the figure of Neoptolemus lies in that he embodies both paradigmatic views as well as the implications of their overcoming: from the epistemological to the moral, from knowing to acknowledging.

Another crucial element in Herder's theory of language is, as mentioned, the central role of hearing and the acoustic. Against the philosophical backdrop of the eighteenth century when the origin of language was considered, first and foremost, to reside in human speech, and specifically, communicative speech concomitant with the constitution of society, Herder's claim conspicuously stands out. The origin of human language in the *Treatise* is not in speech or communication but lies in man's ability to listen. The ear, and not the tongue, marks human beings' entry into language. With this in mind, the relationship between language and pain becomes crucial. Pain is not the object of speech but of hearing; we don't say something about pain but rather hear it. Hearing is therefore the condition of possibility for us to encounter the other's pain in the first place. Moreover, we don't hear our own pain; we hear the pain of others. Similar to Herder's famous example of the sheep's bleating, the cry of pain is not simply understood or confirmed to be expressing a concrete event of affliction; it enters us violently, not leaving any room for doubt or questioning. The cry of pain forces itself on us, something that no propositional claim or linguistic proposition can ever do. This is why Herder describes the sense of hearing as crucial to the constitution of language and the ear as "the organ of language" (*Treatise* 110/*AS* 748).

Heidegger enters the picture at this point in my argument, taking the claim about hearing as his starting point, reflecting on the difference between hearing and listening. However, Heidegger challenges what he considers Herder's limited account of the acoustic grounds of language. In his discussion of what he calls "the crossing-over" (*Übergang*), Heidegger argues that hearing is not merely acoustic but constitutes man's relationship to the world. This relationship is built on the intermediate realm between internal and external, in which the unity of both is ascertained (*Seminar-T* 156/*WS* 190). This has close affinities with Herder: insofar as for him the essence of language is not communicative, at least not in the propositional sense of the word, it also does not originate in an intersubjective domain. This is not to say that for Herder language is not constituted on the grounds of a relationship. Human language originates in the relationship not to another human being but between the human being and the world around him. Language does not represent the world, capturing it with its words and referential structures; nor does the world become an object for humans. Language constitutes man's relation to his world in the first place.

The cry of pain, the structure of sympathy, and the predominance of hearing—the three core constituents of Herder's theory of language—provide us with a clear contestation of the two theoretical paradigms put forth in chapter 1. The cry of pain (its expression as well as its being heard), first, does not destroy language or humanity, and second, does not entail an unbridgeable hiatus between the one suffering pain and those who do not. But the implications of Herder's ideas in the *Treatise* reach much further: they do not merely constitute an alternative, more "positive" way of thinking about the relationship between pain and language. Herder's arguments touch on our conception of the very nature of language itself. This is why Herder' *Treatise on the Origin of Language,* and not simply his claims about language as such, takes such a prominent position in my argument. When we pose the question of the relationship between language and pain together with that of the origin of language, our answer should not merely be given in terms of the characterization of the experience of pain (destructive, isolating) but in those of the nature of language: expression, sympathy, hearing. In other words, posing the problem as though it were limited to the issue of success or failure of an utterance *about* pain keeps out of view a more crucial question: that of the structure of language itself. When we insist on conceiving of language as essentially failing in the face of pain, this relies on the idea that the relationship between the two can only be apprehended as propositional, referential. But language fails only if we treat pain as an internal object, independent of it.

To take the full measure of the alternative view of language I call for here, a consideration of the interrelations between internal and external, in the context of language, is required. Such a perspective takes shape when we observe the strong bond between language and hearing, specifically in the description of the sheep's bleating that enters the soul not as a linguistic sign or representation but as what Herder calls "an internal bleating." But most important, the relationship between internal and external in the context of language emerges when we explore the relationship between language and pain. The understanding of their encounter as a confrontation is grounded in the assumption that pain is an internal, private sensation whereas language is operative by externalizing pain using a propositional structure. Seen this way, language indeed fails.

The alternative, prominently put forth by Wittgenstein, is a rethinking of this hypothesis, undermining the over-conclusive divide between internal and external. The argument I have offered in this chapter suggests that language does not surrender and succumb to this divide or separation but rather constitutes it. Though expression is usually thought of as hingeing on this limit or strict demarcation between inside and outside, according to Hamacher, it is language itself that draws this limit and can therefore not be taken to be subject to it.[8] The claim that language cannot express pain depends on our sometimes limited understanding of the nature of language and the fallacious conception of pain as being engirdled in some unreachable, solipsistic confines being incommensurable with pain. Language is perhaps incapable of "performing" in the face of intense pain, powerless as it is to alter the reality of pain: the perception consequently is that it can barely "touch" pain with its weak, flimsy words.[9]

When we consider language outside of these categories, something else occurs in its encounter with pain: rather than being merely "incapable" of producing a proposition or reference, it is now free from the need to propose and refer. In the face of pain, language stammers, interrupts itself, faces itself, suspended over the abyss of proposition, communication and performance, but it is precisely here that the intimate kinship (not the contradiction!) between language and pain emerges. It is no longer dependent on the success or failure of language's 'performance'; on the contrary, language is established in the confrontation between the experience of intense pain and the essential drive to express, when the former rather than threatening the latter, strengthens it. Contrary to the paradigmatic separation between pain and language, this book takes the challenge of thinking pain and language together, exploring their extraordinary intimacy. To put it differently, if in intense pain, the external world withdraws as an object of reference (and there is nothing but pain), language now relates to pain not as an object but as an experience that is completely internal to it, inseparable from it. It is no longer a language about pain; language now is nothing other than pain itself.

NOTES

Chapter 1

1. Emil M. Cioran, *On the Heights of Despair*, trans. Ilinca Zarifopol-Johnston (University of Chicago Press, 1992): 5.
2. The psychoanalytic tradition is, no doubt, an important resource for the discussion of the relationship between pain and expression. The interconnectedness between pain, suffering, and its expression (verbal or not) has come to be a more or less self-evident presupposition in this perspective (Freud's "talking cure" can be taken as one beginning of this idea). The philosophical perspective on this relationship is, however, less established. My argument seeks to reveal some key moments in the history of philosophy when the kinship between pain and language was not doubted or refuted but given prominence. This is where I abandon the therapeutic perspective on pain, and venture into a philosophical investigation of the problem.
3. Georges Bataille, *Inner Experience*, trans. Leslie Anne Boldt (State University of New York Press, 1988): 72.
4. Emily Dickinson, poem 650 (*The Complete Poems of Emily Dickinson*, ed. Thomas H. Johnson [Little, Brown, 1960]).
5. See also Jean-Luc Marion, *In Excess: Studies of Saturated Phenomena*, trans. Robyn Horner and Vincent Berraud (Fordham University Press, 2002): 92.
6. Freud was concerned with the interconnections between physical and psychic pain as early as his "Project for a Scientific Psychoanalysis" (1895). Despite its importance for the understanding of Freud's overall psychoanalytic project, this work is relatively under-interpreted. A few sources stand out: Valerie D. Greenberg, *Freud and His Aphasia Book* (Cornell University Press, 1997); Anna-Maria Rizzuto, "Freud's Speech Apparatus and Spontaneous Speech," *International Journal of Psycho-Analysis* 74 (1993): 113–127; and the first chapter of John Forrester, *Language and the Origins of Psychoanalysis* (Macmillan, 1980). See also my discussion of Freud's early work on aphasia, a provoking condition insofar as the connection between pain and language is concerned: Ilit Ferber, "A Wound without Pain: Freud on Aphasia," *Naharaim: Journal of German Jewish Literature and Cultural History*, 4 (2010): 133–151, also published in a slightly different version in German as Ilit Ferber, "Aphasie, Trauma und Freuds schmerzlose Wunde," in *Freuds Referenzen*, ed. C. Kirchhoff and G. Scharbert (Kulturverlag Kadmos Berlin, 2012): 145–167.
7. Sigmund Freud, "Inhibitions, Symptoms, Anxiety," *The Standard Edition of the Complete Psychological Works of Sigmund Freud*, vol. 20 (1925–1926), ed. James Strachey (Hogarth Press and the Institute of Psycho-analysis, London, 1959): 171.
8. Sigmund Freud, "On Narcissism: An Introduction," *The Standard Edition*, vol. 14 (1914–1916): 82.
9. Sigmund Freud, *Extracts from the Fliess Papers* ("Draft G: Melancholia"), *The Standard Edition*, vol. 1 (1886–1899): 205–206.

10. Freud returns to the metaphor of pain as a wound in his "Mourning and Melancholia," *The Standard Edition*, vol. 4 (1914–1916): 243–258.
11. See J-B. Pontalis, "On Psychic Pain," in *Frontiers in Psychoanalysis: Between the Dream and Psychic Pain*, trans. Catherine Cullen and Philip Cullen (International Universities Press, 1981): 196.
12. Talal Asad criticizes this view arguing that the stark disjunction between an "agent (representing and asserting himself or herself) or a victim (the passive object of chance or cruelty)" is a common modern, secular view. Instead, he claims: "One can think of pain not merely as a passive state (although it can be just that) but as itself agentive" (Talal Asad, *Formations of the Secular: Christianity, Islam, Modernity* [Stanford University Press, 2003]: 79).
13. Emmanuel Levinas, *Time and the Other*, trans. Richard Cohen (Duquesne University Press, 1987): 69.
14. Emmanuel Levinas, "Useless Suffering," in *Entre nous: On Thinking-of-the-Other*, trans. Michael B. Smith and Barbara Harshav (Columbia University Press, 1998): 91–92.
15. Maurice Blanchot, *The Infinite Conversation*, trans. Susan Hanson (University of Minnesota Press, 2003): 120. See also 44–45, 171–173.
16. Jean Améry, "Torture," in *At the Mind's Limits: Contemplations by a Survivor on Auschwitz and Its Realities*, trans. Sidney Rosenfeld and Stella P. Rosenfeld (Indiana University Press, 1980): 33. See also, "At the Mind's Limits," Ibid.:1–20. On the relationship between language and the solipsism of pain in Améry, seeIlit Ferber, "Pain as Yardstick: Jean Améry," *Journal of French and Francophone Philosophy* 24, no. 3 (2016): 3–16. See also Alphonse Daudet's description of his suffering: "There are no words to express it. . . . Words only come when everything is over, when things have calmed down. They refer only to memory, and are either powerless or untruthful" (Alphonse Daudet, *In the Land of Pain*, trans. Julian Barnes [Knopf, 2003]: 15).
17. On the connection between language and violence, see also Paul Ricoeur, "Violence and Language," in *Political and Social Essays* (Ohio University Press, 1974): 32–41.
18. Virginia Woolf, *On Being Ill: Notes from Sick Rooms* (Paris Press, 2002): 6–7. (quoted in Elaine Scarry, *The Body in Pain: The Making and Unmaking of the World* (Oxford University Press, 1985): 4).
19. Virginia Woolf, *The Waves* (Harvest Books, 1978): 263.
20. An important exception is obviously Ludwig Wittgenstein's *Philosophical Investigations* and his preliminary studies from 1933 to 1935 published in *The Blue and Brown Books*. These two texts mark a turning point in the conception of the relationship between pain and language and were taken on by J. L. Austin and Stanley Cavell. I discuss the latter's interpretation of Wittgenstein in detail in chapter 5.
21. Scarry, *The Body in Pain*. Although her contribution to the study of pain, especially in the context of political thought, cannot be doubted, Scarry was criticized by many. For some of the most perceptive critical accounts, see especially Asad, *Formations of the Secular*: 79–85; Robert M. Cover, "Violence and the Word," *Yale Faculty Scholarship Series*, paper 2708 (1986): 1601–1629; Peter Fitzpatrick, "Why the Law Is Also Nonviolent," in *Law, Violence, and the Possibility of Justice*, ed. Austin Sarat, 142–173 (Princeton University Press, 2001); Lucy Bending, *The Representation of Bodily Pain in Late Nineteenth-Century English Culture* (Oxford University Press, 2000): 82–115.
22. Peter Singer argues that even in the framework of the discussion of torture, Scarry is inaccurate. See his "Unspeakable Acts" (review of E. Scarry, *The Body in Pain: The Making and Unmaking of the World* and E. Peters, *Torture*), *New York Review of Books*, February 27, 1986.
23. Scarry, *The Body in Pain*: 52, 50.
24. Ibid.: 15.
25. Ibid.: 4, 13.
26. Susan Sontag, *Illness as Metaphor* (Ferrar, Straus and Giroux, 1978): 61, 64.
27. Ibid.: 69.
28. Ibid.: 65.
29. Scarry, *The Body in Pain*: 4.
30. Ibid.: 5.

31. Hannah Arendt, *The Human Condition* (University of Chicago Press, 1998): 50–51. See also Arendt's remarks on pain and the experience of its absence in Ibid.: 112–115.
32. Scarry, *The Body in Pain*: 4.
33. Ibid.: 4.
34. Ibid.: 4.
35. Alec Hyslop, *Other Minds* (Kluwer, 1995): 7.
36. Thomas Nagel, *The View from Nowhere* (Oxford University Press, 1986).
37. Peter Smith and O. R. Jones, *The Philosophy of Mind: An Introduction* (Cambridge University Press, 1986): 198–199.
38. There are, no doubt, other cases worth contemplating in this context. One of those would be the traumatic silence of the inability to express one's suffering, when its expression in language poses a deep threat to the psyche. Silence then manifests something of a protective instinct. I take silence about pain, however, to be yet another form of its expression (I discuss this further in chapter 2). Giorgio Agamben's account of the Muselmann is also constructive in this context. For Agamben, the figure of the Muselmann marks a limit between human and inhuman; it also importantly challenges this limit, as his very existence testifies to the fact that it is fundamentally impossible to separate the two. See Agamben, *Remnants of Auschwitz*, trans. Daniel Heller-Roazen (Zone Books, New York, 1999).
39. For an account of the connection between suffering and the constitution of a community see also Maurice Blanchot, *The Unavowable Community* (Station Hill Press, 1988) and Jean-Luc Nancy, *The Inoperative Community* (University of Minnesota Press, 1991).
40. Johann Gottfried Herder, "Treatise on the Origin of Language" [*Abhandlung über den Ursprung der Sprache*], in *Philosophical Writings*, trans. and ed. Michael N. Forster (Cambridge University Press, 2002): 65–164 (hereafter *Treatise*). There are several German editions of the *Treatise*. I am here using the one published in *Werke*: Bd. 1: Frühe Schriften 1764–1772, ed. Urich Gaier (Deutscher Klassiker Verlag, 1985): 697–810 (hereafter *AS*). Herder wrote the *Treatise* in response to the following prize-question announced by the Berlin Academy in 1769: "Supposing men abandoned to their natural faculties, are they in a position to invent language? And by what means will they arrive at this invention?" Herder treats the two parts of the question separately, devoting one part of his essay to each.
41. Michael N. Forster has discussed the important relationship between Herder and Wittgenstein in detail in his "Gods, Animals, and Artists: Some Problem Cases in Herder's Philosophy of Language" (*Inquiry* 46 [2003]: 65–96) and "Herder's Philosophy of Language, Interpretation, and Translation: Three Fundamental Principles" (*Review of Metaphysics* 56, no. 2 [2002]: 323–356). See also Charles Taylor, "The Importance of Herder," in *Isaiah Berlin: A* Celebration, ed. Edna and Ullmann-Margalit and Avishai Margalit (University of Chicago Press, 1991): 40–63.
42. Johann Gottfried Herder, "On Cognition and Sensation of the Human Soul: Observations and Dreams," in *Philosophical Writings*, trans. and ed. Michael N. Forster (Cambridge University Press, 2002): 189 (hereafter *Cognition*). Sophocles appears here in line with Homer, Dante, Shakespeare, and Klopstock.
43. The list is obviously much longer and includes plays, poems, and stories (not to mention artworks). Oscar Mandel's book, *Philoctetes and the Fall of Troy: Documents, Iconography, Interpretations* (University of Nebraska Press, 1981), is an exhaustive source that includes full versions of the story by Sophocles (54–94), Gide (162–178), Müller (222–250), and Mandel himself (185–213). For other versions of the story, see also (to name just a few) Aeschylus and Euripides' versions (only partial fragments survive); Chateaubrun, *Philoctète, tragédie* (1755); Johann Gottfried Herder, "Philoktetes: Scenen mit Gesang" (probably 1774); William Wordsworth, "When Philoctetes in the Lemnian Isle" (1827); Seamus Heaney, *The Cure at Troy: A Version of Sophocles' Philoctetes* (Farrar, Straus and Giroux, 1991). Other more recent versions include Tom Stoppard's television drama *Neutral Ground* (1968), Mark Merlis' novel *An Arrow's Flight* (1999), and James Baxter's play *The Sore-Footed Man* (1967). For a comprehensive list of modern adaptations of the story, see Felix Budelmann, "The Reception of Sophocles' Representation of Physical Pain," *American Journal of Philology* 128, no. 4 (2007): 443–467, and Eric Dugdale, "Philoctetes" in *Brill's Companion to the Reception of Sophocles*, ed. R. Lauriola and K. N. Demetriou (Brill, 2017): 77–145.

44. There are numerous good translations of Sophocles' *Philoctetes*. I am using Hugh Lloyd-Jones' translation published in the Loeb Classical Library series (Harvard University Press, 1998) (bi-lingual edition) (hereafter *Sophocles, Philoc.* with line no).
45. My description here follows Edmund Wilson's account in his "Philoctetes: The Wound and the Bow," in *The Wound and the Bow: Seven Studies in Literature* (Houghton Mifflin Company, Riverside Press, 1941): 272–295.
46. Herder, "Philoktetes: Scenen mit Gesang," in *Nachlaß veröffentlicht, Sämmtliche Werke*. [Abt.] Zur schönen Literatur und Kunst 6. Theil, ed. J. G. Herder (Cotta, 1806): 113–126 (hereafter *Herder, Philoc.*). Since there is no published English translation of this text, all following translations are my own. In certain cases I use Liliane Weissberg's translation of some passages in her "Language's Wound: Herder, Philoctetes, and the Origin of Speech," *Modern Language Notes* 104, no. 3 (1989): 548–579.
47. Thomas Bauman, *North German Opera in the Age of Goethe* (Cambridge University Press, 1985): 152.
48. See Weissberg, "Language's Wound": 576–577.
49. See, for example, Quintus of Smyrna's graphic description of Philoctetes' pain: "So evil suffering overpowered Philoctetes in his wide cavern. His whole body was wasted away; he was nothing but skin and bones. His cheeks were filthily squalid, and he was hideously dirty. Pain beyond curing overwhelmed him, and the eyes of the terribly suffering hero were sunk deep under his brows. He never stopped groaning, because severe pains kept gnawing at the base of his black wound. It had putrefied on the surface and penetrated to the bone" (Mandel, *Philoctetes and the Fall of Troy*: 29). See also Morris' remarks on the unique role of pain in Sophocles' *Philoctetes* in David B. Morris, *The Culture of Pain* (University of California Press, 1993): 248–255.
50. Heiner Müller, "Philoctetes," in *Philoctetes and the Fall of Troy*, trans. Oscar Mandel in collaboration with Maria Kelsen Feder (University of Nebraska Press, 1981): 234(hereafter *Müller, Philoc.*).
51. Sophocles refers to this entanglement: "And he moved this way or that, crawling, like a child without a loving nurse, searching for his need to be supplied, when the plague that devoured his mind abated" (*Sophocles, Philoc.* 700–705, translation altered). Edith Hall contests this argument and claims that according to Greek conceptions of suffering, Philoctetes was not in any way ennobled by his suffering, nor did he learn anything from it. The representation of suffering in the play comes, rather, to raise ethical questions regarding humans' different responses to the suffering of others (in Sophocles we have three such models: Odysseus, the chorus, and Neoptolemus); see Edith Hall, "Ancient Greek Responses to Suffering: Thinking with Philoctetes," in *Perspectives on Human Suffering*, ed. J. Malpas and N. Lickiss (Springer, 2012): 157. See Wilson's renowned account of the story and his emphasis on the inherent link between Philoctetes' disability and his "superior strength" (Wilson, "Philoctetes: The Wound and the Bow": 287).

Chapter 2

1. Some of the other figures Herder criticizes include Condillac, Rousseau, Diodorus Sicilus, and Vitruvius (*Treatise* 76–77/*AS* 710–711).
2. Herder was famously identified by Isaiah Berlin as a Counter-Enlightenment thinker. However, in the last decade, this term has been fiercely challenged and in many cases specifically around Berlin's treatment of Herder. See, for instance, Frederick C. Beiser, "Berlin and the German Counter-Enlightenment," in *Isaiah Berlin's Counter-Enlightenment*, ed. Joseph Mali and Robert Wokler, *Transactions of the American Philosophical Society* 93, no.5 (2003): 105–116; Robert E. Norton, "The Myth of the Counter-Enlightenment," *Journal of the History of Ideas* 68, no. 4 (2007): 635–658. See also Steven Lestition's interesting criticism of Norton in "Countering, Transposing, or Negating the Enlightenment? A Response to Robert Norton," *Journal of the History of Ideas* 6, no. 4 (2007): 659–681, and Norton's reply: "Isaiah Berlin's 'Expressionism,' or 'Ha! Du Bist das Blökende!,'" *Journal of the History of Ideas* 69, no. 2 (2008): 339–347. See an elaborate discussion of this at the end of the chapter.

3. See also the interesting paragraph which ends the *Treatise*. Referring to the treatise's author, namely himself, Herder writes: "How happy he would be if with this treatise he were to displace a hypothesis that, considered from all sides, causes the human soul only fog and dishonor, and moreover has done so for too long! For just this reason he has transgressed the command of the Academy and *supplied no hypothesis*. For what would be the use of having one hypothesis outweigh or counterbalance the other? And how do people usually regard whatever has the form of a hypothesis but as a philosophical novel—*Rousseau's, Condillac's*, and others?" He has preferred to work "at *collecting firm data from the human soul, human organization, the structure of all ancient and savage languages*, and *the whole household-economy of the human species*," and "at *proving* his thesis in the way that the firmest *philosophical truth* can be proved. He therefore believes that with his disobedience he has achieved the will of the Academy more than it could otherwise have been achieved" (*Treatise* 164/*AS* 810).
4. Charles Taylor, Michael N. Forster, and Sonia Sikka are just a few examples. Liliane Weissberg's work stands out. In her excellent "Language's Wound: Herder, Philoctetes, and the Origin of Speech" (*Modern Language Notes* 104, no. 3 [1989]: 548–579), she offers a careful reading of the beginning of Herder's text and elaborates on his use of the figure of Philoctetes in the linguistic as well as aesthetic context. I refer to her article in the following pages.
5. Herder, "Fragments on Recent German Literature" [excerpts on language], in *Philosophical Writings*: 33–64 (hereafter *Fragments*).
6. Herder uses the term *Besonnenheit*, which denotes a combination between reflection and awareness. I discuss this in detail in chapter 3.
7. Herder discusses Süßmilch in the *Treatise* referring mainly to Süßmilch's 1766 *Versuch eines Beweises, daß die erste Sprache ihren Ursprung nicht vom Menschen, sondern allein vom Schöpfer erhalten habe* [Attempt at a Proof that the First Language Received its Origin not from Man but Solely from the Creator] (1766). Süßmilch is also discussed in *Fragments* 55–58.
8. Philoctetes appears only one more time in the *Treatise*, again in a comparison: "This poor earth-dweller comes wretched into the world without knowing that he is wretched; he needs pity without being able to make himself in the least deserving of it; he cries, but even this crying ought to become as burdensome as was the howling of Philoctetes, even though he had so many meritorious accomplishments, to the Greeks, who abandoned him to the desolate island" (*Treatise* 140/*AS* 784).
9. Herder, "Kritische Wälder oder Betrachtungen, die Wissenschaft und Kunst des Schönen betreffend," in *Schriften zur Ästhetik und Literatur, 1767–1781*, ed. Günter E. Grimm, vol. 2 of Johann Gottfried Herder, *Werke* (Frankfurt am Main: Deutscher Klassiker Verlag, 1993): 57–245. Translated as "Critical Forests, or Reflections on the Art and Science of the Beautiful in *Selected Writings on Aesthetics*, ed. and trans. Gregory Moore (Princeton University Press, 2006). In the following I address the two chapters of this text: *First Grove, Dedicated to Mr. Lessing's Laocoön*," in *Selected Writings on Aesthetics*: 51–176 (hereafter *First Grove*); *Fourth Grove, On Riedel's Theory of the Beaux Arts*," in *Selected Writings on Aesthetics*: 177–290 (hereafter *Fourth Grove*). See also Moore's remarks on these texts in *Selected Writings on Aesthetics*: 5–17.
10. Johann Joachim Winckelmann, *Reflections on the Imitation of Greek Works in Painting and Sculpture* [*Gedanken über die Nachahmung der griechischen Werke in der Malerei und Bildhauerkunst*], trans. Henry Fusseli (London, 1765) (hereafter *Reflections*); Gotthold Ephraim Lessing, *Laocoön: An Essay on the Limits of Painting and Poetry* [*Laokoön oder Über die Grenzen der Malerei und Poesie*], trans: Edward Allen McCormick (Johns Hopkins University Press, 1962) (hereafter *Laocoön*).
11. See Gregory Moore, "Introduction," in Herder, *Selected Writings on Aesthetics*: 8.
12. Herder's following explanation of his title is somewhat amusing, yet it also teaches us something important about his philosophical approach in this text: "What are my *Critical Forests*? They were written as chance dictated and more in keeping with my reading than through any systematic development of general principles. They show, however, that we can go astray unsystematically, too, that we can just as easily take a false step not only when we deduce anything we want in the most beautiful order from a few postulated definitions, but also when we do so from several torn-out passages in the most beautiful disorder. . . . For the time being I ask only *one thing*: that the title of my book be not made the object of amusing quibbles,

in which many of the wits among our critics are not found wanting. In more than one language the word *forests* or *silvae* suggests the idea of assembled materials without plan and order; I only hope that my readers shall endure the journey along the somewhat dusty and secluded path of this first part, so that once they have reached its end, they may command clearer views" (*First Grove* 175–176).

13. *Herder, Philoc.*
14. I do not present Herder's texts in the order in which they were written and will therefore begin with the later *Treatise* and then proceed with the earlier *First Grove.*
15. Herder prepares the ground for the unusual opening sentence in his "Fragmente zu einer Archäologie des Morgenlandes" (1769), where he undermines the Cartesian categorical separation between men and animal: "Der Mensch unter den Thieren der Erde! Ein edler Zug der alten Morgenländischen Einfalt! Er, aus Erde gebauet, von der Erde sich nährend, in Erde zerfallend—was ist er, als ein Thier der Erde! . . . Thier unter Thieren! Aber der Mensch ist ein göttlich geadeltes Thier!" [Man among the animals of the earth! A noble deed of ancient Oriental simplicity! He, who was built from earth, nourished from it [earth], disintegrated into earth—what is he but a beast of the earth! . . . Animal among animals! But man is a divine noble animal!] (Suphan-Ausg. Bd. 7, S. 251) (quoted in Wolfgang Proß, *Johann Gottfried Herder, Abhandlung über den Ursprung der Sprache: Text, Materialen, Kommentar* (Carl Hanser Verlag, 1978): 113.
16. Peter Hanly, "Marking Silence: Heidegger and Herder on Word and Origin," *Studies in Christian Philosophy* (*Studia Philosophiae Christianae*) 4 (2013): 74.
17. Friedrich Kittler proposes an interesting reading of the relationship between the "sigh" (*Ach!*) and the sign, that is, between the immediate form of bodily expression and the first signifying word. This argument appears together with his famous dictum in the context of Goethe's Faust, that "German poetry begins with a sigh." He continues: "The sign "oh!" (ach!) is the sign of the unique entity (the soul) that, if it were to utter another signifier or (because signifiers exist only in the plural) any signifier whatsoever, would immediately become its own sigh of self-lament; for then it would have ceased to be soul and have become 'Language' instead" (Kittler, *Discourse Networks 1800/1900*, trans. Michael Metteer with Chris Cullens [Stanford University Press, 1990]: 3. Kittler also points at another interesting and notable fact: the "Ach!" constitutes the middle part of the German word *Sprache* (language) (45).
18. Herder, "On Cognition and Sensation of the Human Soul," in *Philosophical Writings*: 191 (hereafter *Cognition*).
19. For more references to the sounds of Philoctetes' cries before the abandonment, see also *Sophocles, Philoc.* 7–11; *Müller, Philoc.* 223.
20. Emmanuel Levinas, *Time and the Other*, trans. Richard Cohen (Duquesne University Press, 1987): 69 (see a more extensive version of the quote in chapter 1).
21. In *Müller*'s version, Philoctetes tells Neoptolemus that he and the island are named "in one breath" and that he is tied with indestructible chains to the sea surrounding the island: "I, Philoctetes and Lemnos, my island" (*Müller, Philoc.* 231).
22. See also *Müller, Philoc.* 230; Accius' verse: "In dwelling dank, / Where from the dumb walls re-echo piteous sounds of lamentation, plaints and groans and cries" (quoted in Mandel, *Philoctetes and the Fall of Troy*: 38).
23. See also Gide's version in which the kinship between the cry and song is demonstrated: "[Ulysses] Shsh! Listen. . . . Don't you hear something? [Neoptolemus] Yes: the sound of the sea. [Ulysses] No. It's he! His frightful cries are just beginning to reach us. [Neoptolemus] Frightful? On the contrary, Ulysses, I hear singing. [Ulysses] *[listening closely]*. It's true, he is singing. He's a good one! Now that he's alone, he sings! When he was with us, he screamed. [Neoptolemus] What is he singing? [Ulysses] I can't yet make out the words. Listen: he's coming nearer. [Neoptolemus] He has stopped singing. He is standing still. He has seen our tracks in the snow. [Ulysses] *[laughing]*. And now he is beginning to scream again. Ah, Philoctetes! [Neoptolemus] It's true, his cries are horrible" (André Gide, "Philoctetes; or, the Treatise on Three Ethics," in *Philoctetes and the Fall of Troy: Documents, Iconography, Interpretations*, trans. Oscar Mandel, ed. Oscar Mandel [University of Nebraska Press, 1981]: 167) (hereafter *Gide, Philoc.*). I discuss this dialogue below.

24. It is, however, not only when Philoctetes appears on the stage that the vocabulary as well as the performance of sounds, cries, and hearing are so central; they dominate Sophocles' drama throughout. When Odysseus appears before Philoctetes toward the middle of the play, Philoctetes recognizes him by his voice: "Whose voice is that? Did I hear Odysseus?" (*Sophocles, Philoc.* 1295). In Neoptolemus' case, there are two important moments: When he first encounters Philoctetes, the latter first refers to the sound of his speech: "O dearest of sounds! Ah" (234). Then, toward the end of the play, after Neoptolemus has had his change of heart, he returns to Philoctetes' cave in order to make amends. He stands outside the cave, shouting, "What is this clamour of shouting by the cave? Why do you call me out?" (1260), Philoctetes asks; "Listen to the message that I come with!" (1269), answers Neoptolemus.
25. See also *Sophocles, Philoc.* 220–235.
26. Herder, *SW*, Band 2: 924. Quoted in Weissberg, "Language's Wound": 555. The full quote goes as follows: "Ein leidendes Tier, wenn es gleich einsam, verlassen, auf einer wüsten Insel, ohne Anblick, Spur, und Hoffnung eines Hülfreichen Nebengeschöpfs wäre: es wird wimmern! es wird ächzen! es wird mit hohlen, schmerzhaften Klagetönen die ganze Hülflose Gegend erfüllen. . . . So wenig hat uns die Natur als Inseln, als abgesonderte, einzelne Steinfelsen geschaffen! . . . So füllete der Held *Philoktet*, von seinem brennenden unheilbaren Schmerz angefallen, mit Wehklagen das Griechische Lager, wenn er gleich wußte, daß ihn Alle deswegen hasseten und Niemand ihm helfen konnte: Und so füllete er nach seiner Aussetzung das wüßte Eiland, ob gleich keine Spur eines helfenden Wesens um ihn war. Die Empfindung, der Schmerz hat in der ganzen tierischen fühlbaren Natur seine umittelbare Stimme und Sprache, und es ist Eine der falschen Überfeinheiten eines bekannten Philosophen, daß leidende Tiere still und stumm leiden: sie wimmern so gut, als der Mensch, und der Mensch nicht besser als ein Tier."
27. See also *Herder, Philoc.*
28. Weissberg, "Language's Wound": 578.
29. Scarry, *The Body in Pain*: 51.
30. Scarry, *The Body in Pain*: 6.
31. There are many more such allusions. Philoctetes is described, for instance, as "living among beasts in the wilds" (184) and as rending "the air with resounding groans" (or in Meineck and Woodruff's translation: "He's groaning in anguish" [214]). See also Müller's version where Neoptolemus, seeing Philoctetes for the first time, says: "He seems more animal than man. Black vultures swarm above his head" (*Müller, Philoc.* 228).
32. Herder writes about Winckelmann and Lessing that "the former is a sublime master of art; the latter a cheerful companion even in the philosophical passages of his writings, and his book is an entertaining dialogue for our mind. Thus might we describe both men. And how different! How excellent in their differences! So let us be rid of the spectacles through which we squint at them, peering from one to the other in order to praise through contrast! Whoever cannot read L. and W. as they are shall read neither; he shall read only himself!" (*First Grove* 54).
33. For more detailed studies of Lessing's *Laocoön*, see W. J. T. Mitchell, "The Politics of Genre: Space and Time in Lessing's Laocoon," *Representations* 6 (1984): 98–115; David Wellbery, *Lessing's Laocoon: Semiotics and Aesthetics in the Age of Reason* (Cambridge University Press, 1984); Victor Anthony Rudowski, "Lessing Contra Winckelmann," *Journal of Aesthetics and Art Criticism* 44, no. 3 (1986): 235–243; Susan E. Gustafson and McCormick, "Sadomasochism, Mutilation, and Men: Lessing's 'Laokoon,' Herder's 'Kritische Wälder,' Gerstenberg's 'Ugolino,' and the Storm and Stress of Drama," *Poetics Today* 20, no. 2 ("Lessing's Laokoon: Context and Reception") (1999): 197–218.
34. Winckelmann, *Reflections*, quoted in Lessing, *Laocoön*: 7.
35. For obvious reasons, I cannot go into the details of the debate between Lessing and Winckelmann. Let me just state its general outline: Although Lessing agrees with Winckelmann that there is a certain disproportion between Philoctetes' suffering and the intensity of his cry, he locates the reason elsewhere. According to Winckelmann, Philoctetes, as well as other Greek heroes represented in Sophocles' plays, cries out in pain but "do[es] not consider it unmanly to do so." Lessing claims that Philoctetes' relatively subdued cries should be explained aesthetically. That is, according to the laws of beauty in visual arts in antiquity, the ugliness of the screaming open mouth must not be represented; instead, visual art has

to present what Lessing calls the "pregnant moment," a moment that does not represent the peak of the cry but only its potential.

36. Weissberg provides a useful analysis of the differences between the accounts of Winckelmann, Lessing, and Herder, including many details I do not discuss here. She also offers a meticulous account of Herder's various references to Philoctetes. See Weissberg, "Language's Wound": 563ff. See also Gregory Moore, "Introduction," in Herder, *Selected Writings on Aesthetics*: 5–11.
37. Winckelmann, "Winckelmann's Remarks on the Laököon" [passages from *Geschichte der Kunst des Alterthums*], trans. E. S. Morgan, *Journal of Speculative Philosophy* 2, no.4 (1869): 215.
38. For a discussion of this term and its relation to Herder's movement from drama to sculpture, see also Weissberg, "Language's Wound": 564–565.
39. See Weissberg's discussion of Lessing's account of Philoctetes in the context of performed drama in "Language's Wound": 562.
40. This comes up explicitly in the play when Philoctetes tells this story to Neoptolemus, describing his own deed as an act of "kindness" done to Heracles (*Sophocles, Philoc.* 667).
41. Edmund Wilson points out how Philoctetes' superiority (moral and other) is inseparable from his affliction and suffering. There is also a lengthy discussion of this superiority in the context of Philoctetes' ability to bear his pain in the famous debate between Lessing and Winckelmann (Wilson, "Philoctetes: The Wound and the Bow," *The Wound and the Bow: Seven Studies in Literature* [Houghton Mifflin, 1941]: 287–288).
42. For a lengthy discussion of Neoptolemus' moral transformation, see chapter 5.
43. See also Herder's intriguing use of the string metaphor in his description of Homer in *First Grove*: "Every one of Homer's pictures is musical: the tone reverberates in our ears for a little while; if it should begin to fade, the same string is struck and the tone rings out once more, this time with greater force; and all the different tones combine to create the harmony of the picture. In this way, Homer overcomes the principal drawback of his art: that its effect vanishes, as it were, with each passing moment. In this way, he enables each detail of his picture to endure" (*First Grove* 137).
44. Adam Smith, *The Theory of Moral Sentiment*, ed. Knud Haakonssen (Cambridge University Press, 2002), see especially Part 1: 11–35; David Hume, A *Treatise of Human Nature*, ed. D. F. Norton and M. J. Norton (Oxford University Press, 2000), see especially Book 3, Part 2, Sections 7–9: 238–250; Book 3, Part 3, Section 1: 367–378; Jean-Jacques Rousseau, "The Essay on the Origin of Languages in Which Melody and Musical Imitation Are Treated," in *The Discourses and Other Early Political Writings*, trans. and ed. Victor Gourevitch (Cambridge University Press, 1997): 247–299 (hereafter *Essay*), see especially chapters 9–10: 267–280, and "Discourse on the Origin and Foundations of Inequality among Men *or* Second Discourse," in *The Discourses and Other Early Political Writings*: 111–188, see especially Rousseau's discussion of pity on 152–154. For an excellent discussion of sympathy in the theatrical context in Smith and Rousseau, see David Marshall's *The Surprising Effects of Sympathy: Marivaux, Diderot, Rousseau, and Mary Shelley* (Chicago University Press, 1988) and his *The Figure of Theater: Shaftesbury, Defoe, Adam Smith, and George Eliot* (Columbia University Press, 1986).
45. Hume continues by linking this sympathy with an argument regarding the central role of the causal structure in inducing sympathy: "When I see the effects of passion in the voice and gesture of any person, my mind immediately passes from these effects to their causes, and forms such a lively idea of the passion, as is presently converted into the passion itself. . . . No passion of another discovers itself immediately to the mind. We are only sensible of its causes or effects. From these we infer the passion: And consequently these give rise to our sympathy" (*A Treatise of Human Nature*, Book 3, Part 3, Section 1: 368).
46. Proß remarks that Herder's theory of consonance is indebted to the works of Gassendi, Rameau, d'Alembert, and Euler (who were influenced by Leibniz and Newton), as well as by Athanasius Kircher's (1601–1680) "Magnetischen Weltbildes" (see Proß, *J. G. Herder, Abhandlung*: 113).
47. See also Herder's remarks on the sympathetic relation between strings and its connection to emotional effect in *Fourth Grove* 236–243.

48. Herder, *Outlines of a Philosophy of the History of Man*, trans. T. Churchill (Bergman, 1800 [republished in 2016 by Random Shack]): 232–239 (hereafter *Ideas*).
49. Herder develops a similar argument in his writings on history and nationalism when he discusses the differences between the "strings" of different nations and cultures. See, for example, his discussion in *Fourth Grove*: "The sensibility of human nature is not exactly identical in every region of the earth. A different tissue into which the strings of sensation are woven; a different world of objects and sounds that initially rouse one dormant string or another by setting it in motion; different powers that tune one string or another to a different pitch, thereby setting its tone forever, so to speak—in short, there is a quite different arrangement of our faculty of perception, and yet it still lies in the hands of Nature" (*Fourth Grove* 200; see also 247ff).
50. Interestingly, this not only appears in Herder's description of natural, animal sympathy but also when he mentions the "deaf winds" that are filled with the cries of pain, and carry them, spreading them through nature. The winds thereby perform their "natural duty" without a shred of consciousness or intention (see *Treatise*: 65).
51. These "mechanical" depictions of sympathy follow from Herder's repeated descriptions of animals as "sensitive machines" (*empfindenden Maschine*) or "suffering machines" in the treatise (see, for instance, *Treatise* 73, 74, 79, 80/*AS* 705, 706, 713, 715).
52. Agamben's remarks on the relationship between voice, death, and language are interesting in this context. Agamben claims that Herder's *Treatise* was on Hegel's mind when he wrote about animal voice and death. He quotes Hegel on animal voice and then adds: "We may now understand why the articulation of the animal voice gives life to human language and becomes the voice of consciousness. The voice, as expression and memory of the animal's death, is no longer a mere, natural sign that finds its other outside of itself. And although it is not yet meaningful speech, it already contains within itself the power of the negative and of memory. . . . In dying, the animal finds its voice, it exalts the soul in one voice, and, in this act, it expresses and preserves itself *as dead*. Thus, the animal voice is the *voice of death*" (Giorgio Agamben, *Language and Death: The Place of Negativity* [University of Minnesota Press, 2006]: 45).
53. In *Cognition* Herder returns to the metaphor of the string, using it not only to stake his claim about sympathy, but also to establish the primacy of pain. In his discussion of irritation (*Reiz*) he remarks: "Already in animal nature . . . Nature has woven together a thousand little, living strings into a thousandfold fight, into such a manifold touching and resisting; they make themselves shorter and longer with inner force, participate in the play of the muscle, each in its own way" (*Cognition* 189). Interestingly enough, Herder's harmonious characterization of natural sympathy is accompanied by a depiction of the very opposite sensation: pain. The natural ability to feel-for that Herder finds in the feeling of love and in sympathy, stems from "the *single* law which stirred the little fiber with its little glimmering spark of irritation makes itself visible, namely: *Pain*" (*Cognition* 190). Pain makes us contract, resist and recoil, our nerves "flee and shudder" and our "feeling-bud would close up, like the flower in the face of the cold evening breeze" (*Cognition* 202). Herder resorts to the different senses (hearing, taste, smell), referring to examples such as a disharmonious jarring noise, bad taste or an unpleasant smell—all of which are phenomena of "*retreat*, of *resistance*, of *opposition*, as a gentle *floating towards* and *melting away* shows *transition* and *yielding* in the case of pleasant objects" (*Cognition* 202); these are, however, not mere oppositions. Linking between the beautiful and the sublime, Herder suggests an essential kinship between our inclination to retreat into ourselves in the case of the sublime, and our tendency *to float "towards* from out of oneself, with *sympathy* and *communication*" (*Cognition* 202): our "fibers'" ability to extend themselves outward is therefore, essentially bound up with their ability to recoil back into our enclosed, self-contained physique. Michael N. Forster, the translator of the text, points out that Herder uses in his description the German verb *entsetzt sich*, which can be translated as being "appalled" but literally means "moves itself away." Herder here alludes to the Latin *horrere* which combines an original physical sense, "to stand on end, to shudder," with a psychological sense, "to dread" (see *Philosophical Writings*: 202n 17).

54. *Philosophical Writings*: 384. Herder discerns that the internal division of nature has come about through the evolving distinctions between languages, between nations and religions, and also between humans and the rest of nature, which he considers to be the primary division.
55. I discuss this transformation in detail in chapter 5.
56. See chaper 1 for a more detailed discussion of the problem of other minds.
57. See Hegel's interestingly similar description of what he calls "immediate sympathy," which emerges when a "rapport reaches the highest degree of intimacy and strength and consists of the envisioning subject's not only knowing *of* another subject, seeing and sensing it, but of its knowing *within* it, having an *immediate sympathy* with all that happens in respect of this other individual, experiencing its sensations, as its *own*, without paying any direct attention to it. There are some most remarkable instances of this. A French doctor, for example, treated two women who were very fond of one another, and who experienced one another's illnesses when a considerable distance apart" (*Hegel's Philosophy of Subjective Spirit*, vol. 2: Anthropology, trans. and ed. M. J. Petry [D. Reidel, 1978]: 291).
58. Isaiah Berlin, *Vico and Herder: Two Studies in the History of Ideas* (Chatto & Windus, 1976): 153.
59. Charles Taylor, *Hegel* (Cambridge University Press, 1975): 13.
60. Charles Taylor, "The Importance of Herder," in *Isaiah Berlin: A Celebration*, ed. Edna Ullman-Margalit and Avishai Margalit (University of Chicago Press, 1991): 61. A more detailed version of Taylor's ideas is found in his recently published *The Language Animal: The Full Shape of the Human Linguistic Capacity* (Harvard University Press, 2016). Although Herder is not the main figure in the book, he appears at the very start and continues to occupy a principal role in Taylor's discussion, See esp. 9–14, 27–34. See also Taylor's discussion of the dispute between what he calls HHH (Hamann, Herder, Humboldt), and HLC (Hobbes, Locke, Condillac). See esp. 48–50.
61. Taylor, *Hegel*: 17–18.
62. Michael N. Forster, "Herder's Philosophy of Language, Interpretation, and Translation: Three Fundamental Principles," *Review of Metaphysics* 56, no. 2 (2002): 324.
63. Norton in a rigorous, fierce critique of Berlin's notion of the Counter-Enlightenment, writes: "In reality, there was no such thing as the Counter-Enlightenment—as Berlin describes it—at least not during the eighteenth century, and, even if there had been such a thing, Herder would have been at most a curious observer of it, and probably would have vigorously opposed it. Instead, Berlin's notion of the "Counter-Enlightenment" is a myth, a potent fiction to be sure, but a fiction nonetheless. . . . In fact . . . Herder was a fairly typical defender of the Enlightenment aim of achieving human emancipation through the use of reason" (Robert Edward Norton, "The Myth of the Counter-Enlightenment," *Journal of the History of Ideas* 68, no. 4 (2007): 656.
64. Taylor, "The Importance of Herder": 61.
65. Ernst Cassirer, *The Problem of Knowledge: Philosophy, Science and History since Hegel*, trans. William H. Woglom and Charles W. Hendel (Yale University Press, 1950): 223.

Chapter 3

1. Whenever possible, I use a gender neutral expression, however, in most cases I employ the masculine pronoun ("his" and "himself") as a direct reflection of Herder's own language, prevalent in the eighteenth century.
2. See also "Language is invented . . . just as naturally, and as necessarily for the human being, as the human being was a human being" [ebenso natürlich und dem Menschen Mensch notwendig erfunden, als der Mensch ein Mensch war] (*Treatise* 89/*AS* 724).
3. Herder's philosophy of language was interpreted as being "expressive" by two of his most prominent interpreters: Charles Taylor in his "The Importance of Herder," in *Isaiah Berlin: A Celebration*, ed. Edna Ullman-Margalit and Avishai Margalit (University of Chicago Press, 1991): 40–62 and his *Sources of the Self: The Making of the Modern Identity* (Cambridge University Press, 1989): 368–390 as well as Michael N. Forster in his "Gods, Animals, and Artists: Some Problem Cases in Herder's Philosophy of Language," *Inquiry*

46, no. 1 (2003): 65–96 and his "Herder's Philosophy of Language, Interpretation, and Translation: Three Fundamental Principles," *Review of Metaphysics* 56, no. 2 (2002): 323–356.

4. For a comprehensive account of Besonnenheit, see Sonia Sikka, "Herder's Critique of Pure Reason," *Review of Metaphysics* 61, no. 1 (2007): 47–48. Sikka also discusses Herder's positions on the relationship between language and world in a cultural, political context in Sikka, "Herder on the Relation between Language and World," *History of Philosophy Quarterly* 21, no. 2 (2004): 183–200.
5. Herder's idea of life circles has greatly influenced (although never acknowledged) Heidegger's discussion of the difference between the human being, the animal, and the stone that are, accordingly, world-forming, poor in world, and worldless. These three forms of relation to the world can be closely paralleled to Herder's idea of life circles. This important relationship and its implications deserve their own in-depth analysis, which I will not be able to present here. See Part II of Martin Heidegger, *The Fundamental Concepts of Metaphysics: World, Finitude, Solitude,* trans. William Mc Neill and Nicolas Walker (Indiana University Press, 1955): 169–366. See also Giorgio Agamben's discussion of Heidegger's idea of *Umwelt* in his *The Open: Man and Animal,* trans. Kevin Attell (Stanford University Press, 2004): esp. 39–56. Agamben also thoroughly discusses Jakob von Uexküll, yet another influence on Heidegger. See also Uexküll, "A Stroll through the Worlds of Animals and Men: A Picture Book of Invisible Worlds," *Semiotica* 89 no. 3–4 (1992): 319–391.
6. Note Herder's remark about the difference between the animal's and man's relationship to its world. Toward the end of the *Treatise,* in the context of his argument with Rousseau, Herder writes: "Why does this flower belong to the bee that sucks on it? The bee will answer: Because nature made me for this sucking! My *instinct,* which lands on this flower and no other, is dictator enough for me—let it assign me this flower and its garden as my property! And if now we ask the first human being, Who has given you the right to these plants?, then what can he answer but: Nature, which gave me *the taking of awareness* [*Besinnung*]! I have come to know these plants with effort! With effort I have taught my wife and my son to know them! We all live from them! I have more right to them than the bee that hums on them and the cattle that grazes on them, for these have not had all the effort of coming to know and teaching to know!" (*Treatise* 144/*AS* 788).
7. Beiser claims that Herder's portrayal of the life circle is a proto-Darwinian account of why reason, and specifically language, is necessary for the survival of human beings. The extensiveness of their life circle demands that humans master an instrument with which they can convey the conditions of their survival and pass them on to the next generations. Language is therefore an instrument for the storage of information related to humans' life sphere, used as a medium of survival by means of communication (Frederick C. Beiser, *The Fate of Reason: German Philosophy from Kant to Fichte* [Harvard University Press, 1987]: 135).
8. Herder offers an interesting conditional claim, structured in terms of "What if man was an animal?" He thereby proves, within his terms, the necessity of reason (or Besonnenheit) to being human (*Treatise* 84–85/*AS* 719).
9. Similar ideas regarding the superimposition rather than the replacement of emotive language by artificial language appear in different versions in other contemporary thinkers (e.g., Condillac, Diderot, and Rousseau). Compared with those, Herder's originality lies in his successful merging of the emotive and artificial elements of language, as in his use of Besonnenheit. Put differently, Herder's account is important not because he identifies a problem others have failed to notice but because he offers an intricate solution to this problem. In Besonnenheit he finds a way for the two facets to more than coexist: they now productively cooperate.
10. Ludwig Wittgenstein, *Philosophical Investigations,* 4th ed. trans. G. E. M. Anscombe, P. M. S. Hacker, and J. Schulte (Blackwell, 2009), §1: 5e.
11. Ludwig Wittgenstein, *The Brown Book,* in *The Blue and Brown Books: Preliminary Studies for the "Philosophical Investigations"* (Harper & Row, 1960): 157.
12. On the kinship between Herder and Wittgenstein, see esp. Taylor, "The Importance of Herder"; Forster, "Herder's Philosophy of Language, Interpretation, and Translation"; Forster, "Gods, Animals, and Artists."

13. Herder uses the term "flood" also on the first pages of the *Treatise* where he discusses what he calls our "artificial language" that has "dammed, dried out, and drained off the flood and sea of the passions" (*Treatise* 66/*AS* 698–699).
14. On the important role of Herder's Besonnenheit to the evolution of language theories in the eighteenth century and beyond, see Charles Taylor, *The Language Animal: The Full Shape of the Human Linguistic Capacity* (Harvard University Press, 2016): 9–14, 27–34.
15. In *Metacritique of the Critique of Pure Reason*, a much later text, Herder describes this ability when he writes that "in me there is a double 'I'; conscious of myself, I can and must become an object to myself" (quoted in Sonia Sikka, *Herder on Humanity and Cultural Difference: Enlightened Relativism* [Cambridge University Press, 2011]: 163).
16. Dorothea E. von Mücke, *Virtue and the Veil of Illusion: Generic Innovation and the Pedagogical Project in Eighteenth-Century Literature* (Stanford University Press, 1991): 166.
17. See also Ernest Cassirer, *The Philosophy of Symbolic Forms*, vol. 1 (Yale University Press, 1966): 153.
18. Herder presents a different argument in his *Ideas*, where speech features as a condition of being human: "Speech alone awakens slumbering reason: or rather, the bare capacity of reason, that of itself would have remained eternally dead, acquires through speech vital power and efficacy" (*Ideas*, Book 9 76) and further on: "They who are born deaf and dumb, though they may live long in a world of gestures and other characters of ideas, still carry themselves like children, or human animals. They act analogously to what they see, and do not understand; . . . speech alone has rendered man human, by setting bounds to the vast flood of his passions, and giving them rational memorials by means of words" (*Ideas*, Book 9 199–200). Speech and hearing appear inseparable here, similarly to the *Treatise* in which Herder emphasizes time and again that human language is not dependent on the mouth but rather the ear.
19. See also *Treatise* 83, 87ff./*AS* 717, 722ff.
20. Although it is not in the scope of my discussion to elaborate on this point, Herder's somewhat different ideas regarding the essential relationship between language and *Volk* are worth mentioning. See Sonia Sikka, *Herder on Humanity and Cultural Difference* (Cambridge University Press, 2011) and F. M. Barnard, *Herder's Social and Political Thought from Enlightenment to Nationalism* (Clarendon Press, 1967).
21. See Moses Mendelssohn, "Sendschreiben an den Herrn Magister Lessing in Leipzig," in *Gesammelte Schriften Jubiläumsausgabe*, ed. F. Bamberger et al. (Friedrich Fromman Verlag, 1972), vol. 2: 107–108.
22. See von Mücke, *Virtue and the Veil of Illusion*: 298–299, n. 12. On the different critical responses to Rousseau's theory of language, including an account of Mendelssohn's use of the sheep example, see also Avi Lifschitz, *Language and the Enlightenment: The Berlin Debates of the Eighteenth Century* (Oxford University Press, 2012): 82–87.
23. Johann Georg Hamann, "The Last Will and Testament of the Knight of the Rose-Cross," "Philological Ideas and Doubts," and "To the Solomon of Prussia," in *Writings on Philosophy and Language*, ed. and trans. Kenneth Haynes (Cambridge University Press, 2007): 96–110, 111–136, 137–163, respectively. On the relationship between Hamann and Herder, see Daniel O. Dahlstrom, "The Aesthetic Holism of Hamann, Herder and Schiller," in *The Cambridge Companion to German Idealism*, ed. Karl Ameriks (Cambridge University Press, 2017): 76–94 and Katie Terezakis, *The Immanent Word: The Turn to Language in German Philosophy 1759–1801* (Routledge, 2007): esp. chapters 1 and 3.
24. Kant too mentions the human being's relationship to the sheep. However, he presents it completely differently, describing man's instrumental rather than reflective relation to the sheep: "The fourth and last step that reason took in elevating the human being entirely above the society with animals was that he comprehended (however obscurely) that he was the genuine *end of nature*, and that in this nothing that lives on earth can supply a competitor to him. The first time he said to the sheep: *Nature has given you the skin you wear not for you but for me*, then took it off the sheep and put it on himself (Genesis 3: 21), he became aware of a prerogative that he had by his nature over all animals, which he now no longer regarded as his fellow creatures, but rather as means and instruments given over to his will for the attainment of his discretionary aims. This representation includes (however obscurely) the thought of the opposite: that he must not say something like this to any *human being*, but has to regard him

as an equal participant in the gifts of nature—a preparation from afar for the restrictions that reason was to lay on the will in the future in regard to his fellow human beings, and which far more than inclination and love is necessary to the establishment of society" (Immanuel Kant, *Anthropology, History, and Education*, ed. and trans. Robert B. Louden [Cambridge University Press, 2007]: 167).

25. Kittler's reading of this passage foregrounds another interesting element of the scene: "In order for man, this creature of lack and uncertain instincts, to arrive at the freedom of naming, he must lack the instinct of a bloodthirsty line, even that of an ardent ram, both of which might 'throw themselves over' the lamb. . . . If the lamb stands for Woman, then instinct lack posited in Herder's anthropology is simply the cessation of male desire. A desire ceases and the capacity to speak emerges" (Friedrich Kittler, *Discourse Networks 1800/1900*, trans. Michael Metteer with Chris Cullens [Stanford University Press, 1990]: 39). For Kittler, the human lack of instinct not only "purifies" it from distractions, but also, sterilizes it, rendering language a substitute for desire.
26. See Avi Lifschitz, "Language as a Means and an Obstacle to Freedom: The Case of Moses Mendelssohn," in *Freedom and the Construction of Europe*, ed. Quentin Skinner and Martin van Gelderen (Cambridge University Press, 2013): vol. 2, 89–90.
27. The following question, nevertheless, remains open: Is the human being's desire to be "acquainted" with the sheep, instinctual? Herder does not address this explicitly.
28. Smell is an interesting counter case but Herder does not address it.
29. I am indebted to Werner Hamacher for our conversations regarding this point.
30. Forster explains that the word *werde* can be understood in an epistemic as well as a developmental sense (*Treatise* 132n. 145).
31. Herder, "Über die Fähigkeit zu sprechen und zu hören," Aus der "Neuen Deutschen Monatsschrift" (1795), *Gesammelte Abhandlungen, Aufsätze, Beurtheilungen und Vorreden aus der Weimarer Zeit*, Kapitel 17 (G. Hempel, 1897): 174.
32. See my discussion of Herder's idea of the law of nature in chapter 2.
33. David Wellbery, *The Specular Moment: Goethe's Early Lyric and the Beginnings of Romanticism* (Stanford University Press, 1996): 189.
34. Ibid.
35. See note 18, this chapter; Churchill has translated *Ideen* into "Outlines"; however, I prefer to use *Ideas*, which is closer to the German.
36. "Concent" in original.
37. See also Herder's interesting remarks about the relationship between song and speech in *Fragments* 61–63.
38. Martin Heidegger, "What Are Poets For?" *Poetry, Language, Thought*, trans. Albert Hofstadter (Harper Perennial, 2001): 136–137.
39. I am quoting from Albert Hofstadter's translation of these verses as it appears in Heidegger, *Poetry, Language, Thought*. Barnstone's slightly different translation is "True singing is a different breath" (Rainer Maria Rilke, *Sonnets to Orpheus*, trans. Willis Barnstone (Shambhala, 2004): Part I, Sonnet no. 3: 107).
40. Heidegger, "What Are Poets For?": 137.
41. Ibid.: 135.
42. Herder discusses the sense of hearing in *Fourth Grove* and in the *Treatise*. In the former he insists that there is no clear hierarchy between the three senses under discussion (vision, hearing, and touch), whereas in the latter he strongly argues for the primacy of hearing as the "middle sense" and more importantly, the "sense of language."
43. See also Herder's somewhat different comparison between seeing and hearing in the context of his discussion of Lessing: "That which the eye takes in at a single glance, he [the author of a textbook on botany] counts out to us with perceptible slowness, and it often happens that when we arrive at the end of his description we have already forgotten the first features. And yet we are supposed to form a notion of the whole from these features. To the eye, parts once seen remain continually present; it can run over them again and again. For the ear, however, the parts once heard are lost unless they remain in the memory. And if they do remain there, what trouble and effort it costs to renew all their impressions in the same order and with the same vividness; to review them in the mind all at once with only moderate rapidity, to arrive

at an approximate idea of the whole! It may be very nice to recite such descriptions, holding the flower in one's hands; but by themselves they say little or nothing" (*First Grove* 143).

44. *Treatise* 111n98.
45. See also Rachel Zuckert's discussion of Herder's comparison between the senses in the context of his account of sculpture: Zuckert, "Sculpture and Touch: Herder's Aesthetics of Sculpture," *Journal of Aesthetics and Art Criticism* 67, no. 3 (2009): 285–299.
46. *Fourth Grove* 249–250. See also *Fourth Grove* 206–211.
47. Peter Hanly, "Marking Silence: Heidegger and Herder on Word and Origin," *Studies in Christian Philosophy* (*Studia Philosophiae Christianae*) 4 (2013): 79.
48. Jürgen Trabant, "Herder's Discovery of the Ear," *Herder Today: Contributions from the International Herder Conference*, ed. Kurt Mueller-Vollmer (De Gruyter 1990): 358.
49. Ibid.: 356.
50. Ibid.: 359.
51. See my detailed discussion of Herder's first part of the *Treatise* Reason in the context of pain and sympathy in chapter 2.
52. Kittler suggests that the reappearance of the sheep can be read in light of Derrida's *différance* (Kittler, *Discourse Networks*: 40).
53. Kelly Oliver, *Animal Lessons: How They Teach Us to Be Human* (Columbia University Press, 2009): 89.
54. With this argument, I open the way to a rethinking of the relationship between Herder and Heidegger, specifically with regard to Heidegger's idea of Dasein's being-in-the-world (in his early writings), as well as his conception of language (in the later writings). I develop the discussion of this important, productive relationship in chapter 4.
55. See also *Treatise* 94–95/*AS* 730–731 for a longer account of Rousseau's argument, which Herder sarcastically refutes, step by step.
56. See also *Fragments* 60–61, where Herder provides an account very close to Rousseau's state of nature. See also Nigel DeSouza, "Language, Reason, and Sociability: Herder's Critique of Rousseau," *Intellectual History Review* 22, no. 2 (2012): 221–240.
57. Jean-Jacques Rousseau, "Discourse on the Origin and Foundation of Inequality among Men *or* Second Discourse," in *The Discourses and other Early Political Writings*, trans. and ed. Victor Gourevitch (Cambridge University Press, 1997) (hereafter *Discourse*).
58. Jean-Jacques Rousseau, *Emile or on Education*, trans. Alan Bloom (Basic Books, 1979) (hereafter *Emile*).
59. Roueesau, *Essay*.
60. On Herder's criticism of Rousseau see Nigel DeSouza, "Language, Reason, and Sociability: Herder's Critique of Rousseau."
61. See also Rousseau, "Examination of Two Principles Advanced by M. Rameau in His Brochure Entitled: 'Errors on Music in the Encyclopedia,'" in *Essay on the Origin of Languages and Writings Related to Music*, trans. and ed. John T. Scott (University Press of New England, 1988): 747.
62. It is interesting to compare Rousseau's description with Herder's remarks on the newborn child. Comparing human and animal in the *Treatise*, Herder writes: "With each animal, as we have seen, its language is an expression of such strong sensuous representations that these become drives. Hence language is, along with senses and representations and drives, *innate* and *immediately natural* for the animal. . . . But *how does the human being speak by nature? Not at all!*—just as he does little or nothing through sheer instinct as an animal. I make an exception in the case of a newborn child of the cry of its sensitive machine; otherwise *this child is dumb*; it expresses neither representations nor drives through sounds, as by contrast every animal does according to its kind; merely set among animals, therefore, it is the most orphaned child of nature. Naked and bare, weak and needy, timid and unarmed—and, what constitutes the culmination of its miserable state, deprived of all nurturing guides in life. Born with such a dispersed, weakened sensuality, with such indeterminate, dormant abilities, with such divided and weakened drives, obviously dependent on and directed to a thousand needs, destined for a large sphere—and yet so orphaned and abandoned that it does not even enjoy the gift of a language with which to express its shortcomings. . . . No! Such a contradiction is not nature's way of organizing her household. There must, instead of instincts, be other hidden powers sleeping in the human child! *Born dumb*, but . . ." (*Treatise* 80–81/*AS* 715).

63. A similar idea appears in Rousseau's discussion of the word "misery" in the *Second Discourse*. There he argues that savage man in the state of nature is not at all miserable as we tend to think; quite the opposite: "I should very much like to have it explained to me," Rousseau writes, "what kind of misery there can be for a free being, whose heart is at peace, and body in health. I ask, which of the two, Civil life or natural life, is more liable to become intolerable to those who enjoy it? . . . Nothing, on the contrary, would have been as miserable as Savage man dazzled by Enlightenment, tormented by Passions, and reasoning about a state different from his own" (*Discourse* 149–150).
64. Note that in Rousseau's case, contra to Herder, the origin of linguistic expression is not only inaugurated by pain and suffering but emerges specifically when the communication with other human beings becomes necessary. Rousseau explains that "the discomfort of the needs is expressed by signs when another's help is necessary to provide for them. This is the source of children's screams. . . . When they are painful, children say so in their language and ask for relief" (*Emile* 64–65).
65. Giorgio Agamben, *Infancy and History: On the Destruction of Experience*, trans. Liz Heron (Verso, 2007): 48.
66. Leland de la Durantaye, *Giorgio Agamben: A Critical Introduction* (Stanford University Press, 2009): 90–91.
67. Quoted in Agamben, *Infancy and History*: 49.
68. A possible implication of this would be that language no longer has room for the intensity of feeling, so that the existence of language not only mollifies pain, but perhaps even prevents it from being intensively felt in the first place.
69. The similarity to Wittgenstein here is striking. In his *Philosophical Investigations* Wittgenstein discusses the problem of the connection between words and sensations, giving the example of pain. "So you are saying that the word 'pain' really means crying?" asks the interlocutor. "On the contrary," Wittgenstein replies, "the verbal expression of pain replaces crying, it does not describe it. How can I even attempt to interpose language between the expression of pain and the pain?" (Wittgenstein, *Philosophical Investigations*, §244–245: 95e).
70. In a similar context, see also Walter Benjamin's interesting comparison between pain and pleasure in his "Outline of the Psychophysical Problem" (1922–1923), in *Selected Writings*, trans. Rodney Livingstone, ed. Marcus Bullock and Michael W. Jennings, vol. 1, 1913–1926 (Harvard University Press, 1996): 393–401. I have discussed this text as well as Benjamin's thoughts about pain in Ilit Ferber, "'Schmerz war ein Staudamm': Benjamin on Pain," *Benjamin-Studien* 3 (2014): 165–177.
71. Rousseau gives an interesting, yet somewhat different account in the *Discourse* when he links between passion and desire, on one hand, and thought and the emergence of language, on the other: "We seek to know only because we desire to enjoy," he writes, "and it is not possible to conceive why someone who had neither desires nor fears would take the trouble to reason" (*Discourse* 142).
72. See also, Eli Friedlander, *J. J. Rousseau: An Afterlife of Words* (Harvard University Press, 2004): 48–50. Note that in Rousseau's account, the strength of passion is markedly connected with the fact that this is the savage's first *social* encounter.
73. Ibid.: 48.
74. Ibid.: 49.
75. Jacques Derrida, *Of Grammatology*, trans. G. C. Spivak (Johns Hopkins University Press, 1997): 275–280.
76. Derrida, *Of Grammatology*: 275–276.
77. Derrida, *Of Grammatology*: 276.
78. Paul de Man discusses Derrida's interpretation of Rousseau's *Essay* in two main texts: "The Rhetoric of Blindness: Jacques Derrida's Reading of Rousseau," in *Blindness and Insight: Essays in the Rhetoric of Contemporary Criticism* (Oxford University Press, 1971):102–141, and *Allegories of Reading: Figural Language in Rousseau, Nietzsche, Rilke, and Proust* (Yale University Press, 1979): 135–159. As Rei Terada has meticulously proven, these two versions vary in some important points. Since these differences are outside the scope of my discussion, I will briefly present only the second, later text. See Rei Terada, *Feeling in Theory: Emotion after the "Death of the Subject"* (Harvard University Press, 2001), esp. 48–89.

79. De Man, "The Rhetoric of Blindness": 139–140.
80. De Man, *Allegories of Reading*: 151.
81. Ibid.: 150. See also Terada's explanation on the difference between de Man's two texts regarding this point in her *Feeling in Theory*: 56–57.
82. De Man, *Allegories of Reading*: 151.
83. Ibid.: 150.
84. Although de Man adopts a fairly critical tone in his reading of Derrida, his own alternative is grounded, to a large extent, on Derrida's own claims. This is especially true for affinity between Derrida's idea of "inadequacy" and de Man's "indeterminacy," as well as their resemblance insofar as the role of the metaphor is concerned. See Terada, *Feeling in Theory*: esp. 56–58.
85. Gerald L. Bruns, "Language, Pain and Fear," *Iowa Review* 11, no. 2/3 (1980): 131.

Chapter 4

1. Martin Heidegger, *On the Essence of Language: The Metaphysics of Language and the Essencing of the Word. Concerning Herder's Treatise on the Origin of Language*, trans. Wanda Torres Gregory and Yvonna Unna (State University of New York Press, 2004) (hereafter *Seminar* followed by *N* for Heidegger's own notes, and *T* for the student transcripts). The German edition of the *Seminar, Vom Wesen der Sprache: Die Metaphysik der Sprache und die Wesung des Wortes. Zu Herders Abhandlung "Über den Ursprung der Sprache"* was published in vol. 85 of Heidegger's *Gesamtausgabe*, ed. Ingrid Schüßler (Vittorio Klostermann GmbH, 1999) (hereafter *WS*).
2. Insofar as the historical context of Germany is concerned together with the development of Heidegger's own thought and political positions—there is an interesting question as to why he chose to teach Herder in 1939 (a period in which he was occupied with thinkers such as Nietzsche and Schiller). Another puzzle is the fact that in the context of German thought, Herder is no doubt one of the first thinkers of the *Volk*. It is intriguing to wonder why Heidegger did not address this concept in Herder's work and chose, rather, his reflections on language. His silence about *Volk*, is worth contemplating, but this lies outside my scope here.
3. Heidegger, *Contributions to Philosophy (From Enowning)*, trans. Parvis Emad and Kenneth Maly (Bloomington: Indiana University Press, 1999) (hereafter *Contributions*, German pagination in brackets).
4. Heidegger, "*Besinnung*," GA 66, 423, quoted in Ingrid Schüßler, "Editor's Epilogue," *Seminar*, 177.
5. My turn to Heidegger in this chapter neither aims to provide an interpretation of the *Seminar* (which is, in fact, strikingly absent from the secondary literature about Heidegger), nor does it center on establishing an argument regarding Herder's influence on Heidegger (which is strong, no doubt). The *Seminar* is important to me first because Heidegger's analysis of the *Treatise* puts to the fore and illuminates some of the claims that are crucial to my own investigation of Herder. More important, by pointing out some of the lacunas in Herder's position, Heidegger offers an interesting criticism as well as a novel entry point into the rethinking of Herder's *Treatise*.
6. Sonia Sikka, *Herder on Humanity and Cultural Difference: Enlightened Relativism* (Cambridge University Press, 2011): 184, n. 11. The relationship between Heidegger and Herder has not taken a central place in the literature, to say the least. There are, however, two important interpreters who discuss it. The first is Sikka, who discusses it in various studies, especially in her *Herder on Humanity*, and "Heidegger's Concept of Volk," *Philosophical Forum* 26, no. 2 (1994): 101–126. The second is Charles Taylor, who presents a detailed, rigorous discussion of the similarities between Heidegger's and Herder's theories of language; see Taylor, "Heidegger, Language, and Ecology," in *Philosophical Arguments* (Harvard University Press, 1995): 100–126. None of these discussions, however, focus on the *Seminar*, which is rarely dealt with in the secondary literature on Heidegger. George Kovacs is an exception. In his "Heidegger in Dialogue with Herder: Crossing the Language of Metaphysics toward Be-ing-historical Language" (*Heidegger Studies* 17 [2001]: 45–63), he offers a detailed discussion of the *Seminar* focusing on Heidegger's critique of Herder's language of metaphysics. Another source is Kelly Oliver's short discussion of Heidegger's interpretation of Herder in her *Animal Lessons: How They Teach Us to Be Human* (Columbia University Press, 2009): 90–93.
7. See also Martin Heidegger, "Letter on 'Humanism,'" *Pathmarks*, ed.William McNeill, trans. Frank A. Capuzzi (Cambridge University Press, 1998): 239–276.

8. Heidegger, *Being and Time*, trans. Joan Stambaugh (State University of New York Press, 1992) (hereafter *BT*, German pagination in brackets).
9. Considering Heidegger's later philosophy, a crucial difference comes into view: in the *Seminar* (1939), Heidegger is still preoccupied with the problem of the human being, the *linguistic* human being. In his "Language" (1950), to take one prominent example, his interest has already shifted: language and speech are not merely "an activity of man"; rather, language itself speaks and "first brings man about, brings him into existence. Understood in this way, man would be bespoken by language" (Heidegger, "Language," in *Poetry, Language, Thought*: 190).
10. See Martin Heidegger, *Contributions to Philosophy (of the Event)*, trans. Richard Rojcewicz and Daniela Vallega-Neu (Indiana University Press, 2012) and Martin Heidegger, *Nietzsche: Volumes I and II*, trans. David Farrell Krell (Harper & Row, 1979). Another interesting reference point to the term *Übergang*, is no doubt Immanuel Kant, with whose work Heidegger was intimately familiar. On Kant's use of the term see Peter Fenves, *Late Kant: Towards Another Law of the Earth* (Routledge, 2003): 154–170.
11. I am thankful to Peter Fenves for pointing out this problem in translation to me. Another interesting reference point is Heidegger's letter to Ernst Jünger's On "Crossing the Line" ["*Über 'die Linie'*"], which was later published under the title "On the Question of Being" ["*Zur Seinsfrage*"] (Heidegger, *Pathmarks*: 291–322. Although Heidegger does not use *Übergang* there, but rather *Überqueren*, there are, nevertheless some important claims here that are also pertinent to the *Seminar*'s "crossing-over." Briefly stated, Jünger discusses nihilism and the possibility to overcome it by way of crossing its line in a new era in which nihilism is no longer unfulfilled. Heidegger, on the other hand, emphasizes the line itself, rather than the implications of its crossing. As William McNeill sums it up: "In the end, Heidegger argues against Jünger that nihilism cannot be overcome at all and that the question of nihilism must be brought back to the question of Being" (McNeill's foreword to "The Question of Being," in *Pathmarks*: 291, my italics. Cf. Vincent Blok, "An Indication of Being—Reflections on Heidegger's Engagement with Ernst Jünger," *Journal of the British Society for Phenomenology* 42, no. 2 (2011): 194–208.
12. Heidegger's account of the crossing-over appears in the text together with his analysis of three of Stefan George's poems, all of which touch in one way or another on hearing and/or sound ("Sea Song," "The Word," and "Listen to What the Somber Earth Speaks") (*Seminar-N* 51–62/*WS* 61–72).
13. In §13 Heidegger provides the following sketch:

to notice [*merken*]—	to sense, to perceive
to attend to [*aufmerken*]—	to turn oneself towards, to stay with, waiting anxiously, lurking
to note [*be-merken*]—	*to preview—overview*, "free"
to de-mark [*ab-merken*] →	to firmly grasp sign
to retain [*sich merken*]—	← to keep mark, to store, to register, to note down
to note down [*vermerken*]—	to hold fast in a mark
to make noticeable [*bemerkbar machen*]—	to make known.
Mark [*Merkmal*]—	→
	note, notio, nota, character-istic [*Kenn-zeichen*], *fixing of the permanent and always constant in itself* [Festmachen des Beständigen und auf sich je Ständigen]; To differentiate [*merken*]: to ac-knowledge oneself [*An-wesen lassen*] in a differentiating manner

ad—perception ←---→	ad—sensus "oneself"—"saying"!

to notice: as letting pre-sence, to make-present, *retainable* through *"signs"*.

(*Seminar-N* 15/*WS* 18)

14. See also Heidegger's following remarks on taking notice and attention: "Heedfulness [from *Aufmerken*, "noticing," "marking down"]: mark—"sign." The mark—that by which something "emerges" for us, by which we "notice" something, i.e., experience it, i.e., are struck by it, feel its presence; become aware of [*innewerden*]—(intimacy) (these relations more essential than all merely rational "signs"). To notice—*no- tare, animadvertere, memoria tenere, observare, attendere.* Attend to, attentiveness, attention. Keeping in mind. *Marking—consideratio*" (Heidegger, *The Event*, trans. Richard Rojcewicz [Indiana University Press, 2013]: 251–252 [289–290]).
15. See also Heidegger's remarks on hearing and hearkening in *BT* 155–161 [160–167].
16. Heidegger, *Introduction to Metaphysics*, trans. Gregory Fried and Richard Polt (Yale University Press, 2000) (hereafter *IM*, German pagination in square brackets).
17. Heidegger, "Logos (Heraclitus, Fragment B 50)," *Early Greek Thinking: The Dawn of Western Philosophy*, trans. David Farrell Krell and Frank A. Capuzzi (Harper & Row, 1984): 59–78 (hereafter *Logos*).
18. Heidegger, *Bremen and Freiburg Lectures: Insight into That Which Is* and *Basic Principles of Thinking*, trans. Andrew J. Mitchell (Indiana University Press, 2012): 144–166.
19. Heidegger and Eugen Fink, *Heraclitus Seminar 1966/67*, trans. Charles H. Seibert (University of Alabama Press, 1979) (hereafter *Heraclitus*).
20. See also Michael Inwood, *A Heidegger Dictionary* (Blackwell, 1999): 21–22.
21. On hearing, gathering and belonging see also Jacques Derrida, "Heidegger's Ear," ed. John Sallis, *Remembering Heidegger: Commemorations* (Indiana University Press, 1993): esp. 187–193.
22. Already in 1925 Heidegger argues similarly, that when we say of someone that he "cannot hear" (in the case that there is no physiological reason that prevents him from hearing), he may very well be able to hearken. See Heidegger, *History of the Concept of Time: Prolegomena*, trans. Theodore Kisiel (Indiana University Press, 1985): 267 (hereafter *HT*, German pagination in square brackets).
23. Matthew Meyer, "Reflective Listening in Heraclitus," *International Journal of Listening* 21, no. 1 (2007): 60.
24. Heidegger and Fink have an interesting discussion on the relationship between seeing, hearing, and touching. To recall, a detailed comparison between these three senses is at the center of Herder's discussion of the sense of hearing; see chapter 3.
25. Heidegger, *Bremen and Freiburg Lectures*: 152.
26. See also Blanchot's interesting remarks on the role hearing plays for Heidegger, in Maurice Blanchot, *The Infinite Conversation*, trans. Susan Hanson (University of Minnesota Press, 1993): 439–440 n 3.
27. See also the following remark from *Introduction to Metaphysics*: "Gathering is never just driving together and piling up. It maintains in a belonging-together that which contends and strives in confrontation. It does not allow it to decay into mere dispersion and what is simply cast down. As maintaining, *logos* has the character of pervasive sway, of *phusis*. It does not dissolve what it pervades into an empty lack of opposites; instead, by unifying what contends, the gathering maintains it in the highest acuteness of its tension" (*IM* 142–143 [102]).
28. See also *Seminar-T* 133/*WS* 155–156.
29. Derrida, "Heidegger's Ear": 173. See also 178, 185.
30. Heidegger, *BT* 153 [163].
31. Derrida, "Heidegger's Ear": 163–164.
32. Ibid.: 164.
33. Walter Brogan, "Listening to the Silence: Reticence and the Call of Conscience in Heidegger's Philosophy," in *Heidegger and Language*, ed. Jeffrey Powel (Indiana University Press, 2013): 35.
34. For an interesting discussion of the relationship between the authentic and the personal in Heidegger, see Hagi Kenaan, *The Present Personal: Philosophy and the Hidden Face of Language* (Columbia University Press, 2004): 97–102.
35. Brogan, "Listening to the Silence": 37.
36. Proß remarks that Herder's theory of consonance is indebted to the works of Gassendi, Rameau, d'Alembert, and Euler (who in turn are influenced by Leibniz and Newton), as well

as to that of Athanasius Kircher's (1601–1680) "Magnetischen Weltbildes" (see Proß, J. G. Herder, *Abhandlung*: 113).

37. C. S. Lewis, *The Problem of Pain* (Harper Collins, 2015): 91.
38. See Vetlesen's discussion of Merleau-Ponty's similar ideas on pain and the body: Arne Johan Vetlesen, *A Philosophy of Pain*, trans. John Irons (Reaktion Books, 2009): 53–54.
39. I have used this expression as a title to an article about Jean Améry and his experience of torture. See Ilit Ferber, "Pain as Yardstick: Jean Améry," *Journal of French and Francophone Philosophy* 24, no. 3 (2016): 3–16.
40. Marion, *In Excess: Studies of Saturated Phenomena*, trans. Robyn Horner and Vincent Berraud (Fordham University Press, 2002): 92.
41. See also chapter 3.
42. Notwithstanding the similarities between pain and Besonnenheit (attention as well as reflection), there is an interesting difference. Although Besonnenheit too is described as an experience involving the violent separation of the wave (so as to turn it into a *Merkmal*), it is not described as a violent act—at least, there is no violence directed toward the human being. On the contrary, there is even something calm about the "collectedness" Herder refers to. Violence, or that which cannot be opposed or fought, appears elsewhere in the *Treatise* in the paragraphs in which Herder speaks of the way in which the "violent passions" of the soul "announce themselves" violently, claiming their right to speak in their "mother tongue"; this occurs when the language of nature "reassumes its right," in Herder's words. It is, we could say, a violence between the two languages, struggling for primacy.
43. Heidegger has a similar argument in "On the Way to Language"; See Martin Heidegger, *On the Way to Language*, trans. Peter D. Hertz (Harper & Row, 1971): 181.
44. Heidegger, "Language": 201.
45. Ibid.: 201–202.
46. Andrew J. Mitchell, "Entering the World of Pain: Heidegger," *Telos* 150 (2010): 86.
47. Peter Hanly, "Dark Celebration: Heidegger's Silent Music," in *Heidegger and Language*, ed. Jeffrey Powel (Indiana University Press, 2013), 259.
48. Heidegger, "On the Question of Being": 305.

Chapter 5

1. I tell the story of Philoctetes in detail in chapter 1.
2. Full quotes from the *Treatise* are as follows: "A suffering animal, as much as the hero Philoctetes, when overcome with pain, will whine!, will groan!, even if it were abandoned, on a desolate island, without the sight, the trace, or the hope of a helpful fellow creature" (*Treatise* 65/*AS* 697); "This poor earth-dweller comes wretched into the world without knowing that he is wretched; he needs pity without being able to make himself in the least deserving of it; he cries, but even this crying ought to become as burdensome as was the howling of Philoctetes, even though he had so many meritorious accomplishments, to the Greeks, who abandoned him to the desolate island" (*Treatise* 140/*AS* 784). Herder mentions Philoctetes (usually as an example) in several other texts including "This Too a Philosophy of History for the Formation of Humanity [*Auch eine Philosophie der Geschichte zur Bildung der Menschheit*]" (1774) (In *Philosophical Writings*, trans. and ed. Michael N. Forster (Cambridge University Press, 2002) and *Sculpture: Some Observations on Shape and Form from Pygmalion's Creative Dream* [*Plastik: Einige Wahrnehmungen über Form und Gestalt aus Pygmalions bildendem Traume*] (1778), trans. Jason Gaiger (University of Chicago Press, 2002): 57–58.
3. Scarry, *The Body in Pain*: 35.
4. Ibid.: 3, 4.
5. David B. Morris mentions two other scenes in Greek and Renaissance English tragedy in which, at the height of their suffering, heroes can no longer speak in articulate, descriptive sentences and only cry. He refers to Oedipus' cry of agony at the end of *Oedipus Tyrannus*: "When Oedipus finally speaks, what we hear is not words but only a single, repeated cry of agony: speech rolled back into mere sound and torment." The second tragic hero is King Lear who, at the very end of the play enters the stage with the body of dead Cordelia

in his arms, repeating three words in a manner that mimics animal cries: "Howl, howl, howl" (David B. Morris, *The Culture of Pain* [University of California Press, 1993]: 284).

6. Seamus Heaney, *The Cure at Troy: A Version of Sophocles' Philoctetes* (Farrar, Straus and Giroux, 1991): 41.
7. Edith Hall, "Ancient Greek Responses to Suffering: Thinking with Philoctetes," in *Perspectives on Human Suffering*, ed. Jeff Malpas and Norelle Lickiss (Springer, 2012): 163.
8. Bernard M. W. Knox, *The Heroic Temper: Studies in Sophoclean Tragedy* (University of California Press, 1983): 131.
9. Knox, *The Heroic Temper*: 131. See also J. Ceri Stephens, "The Wound of Philoctetes," *Mnemosyne* 48 (1995): 153–168.
10. Felix Budelmann, "The Reception of Sophocles' Representation of Physical Pain," *American Journal of Philology* 128, no. 4 (2007): 445.
11. Hagi Kenaan, *The Present Personal: Philosophy and the Hidden Face of Language* (Columbia University Press, 2005): 8–9.
12. See also Thomas Nagel, *The View from Nowhere* (Oxford University Press, 1986).
13. See also my more elaborate discussion of this problem in chapter 1.
14. Rebecca Comay, "Paradoxes of Lament: Benjamin and Hamlet," in *Lament in Jewish Thought: Philosophical, Theological, and Literary Perspectives*, ed. Ilit Ferber and Paula Schwebel (De Gruyter, 2014): 258–259.
15. Stanley Cavell, "Comments on Veena Das's Essay 'Language and Body: Transactions in the Construction of Pain,'" *Daedalus* 125, no. 1 (1996): 95.
16. Stanley Cavell, *The Claim of Reason: Wittgenstein, Skepticism, Morality, and Tragedy* (Oxford University Press, 1999): 35.
17. Michael N. Forster has written extensively about the relationship between Herder and Wittgenstein. See especially his "Gods, Animals, and Artists: Some Problem Cases in Herder's Philosophy of Language" (*Inquiry* 46 [2003]: 65–96) and "Herder's Philosophy of Language, Interpretation, and Translation: Three Fundamental Principles" (*Review of Metaphysics* 56, no. 2 [2002]: 323–356).
18. Ludwig Wittgenstein, *Philosophical Investigations*, 4th ed., trans. G. E. M. Anscombe, P. M. S. Hacker, and J. Schulte (Blackwell, 2009): §244.
19. Wittgenstein, *Philosophical Investigations*: §245.
20. The story of the beetle-box Wittgenstein sketches in §293 demonstrates this clearly (Wittgenstein uses this parable to make the point that we cannot "know" another's pain through knowledge of our own pain). Suppose we all have boxes with something in them, which we call "beetle." The content of everyone's box is principally inaccessible: I can only know what my "beetle" means, but can never know for certain whether the other "beetles" are the same object as my own. Moreover, the "beetle" can even mean nothing, or emptiness, or an ever-changing object. The point of the beetle-box parable is to show that no matter which way we look at it, the existence of the beetle itself, as a thing, becomes irrelevant and meaningless. The question of its existence thus parallels the adult's inability to "prove" the existence of the child's pain. The content of the box, as well as the child's sensation, resides outside the discussion. Wittgenstein concludes by saying: "If we construe the grammar of the expression of sensation on the model of 'object and designation' the object drops out of consideration as irrelevant" (Wittgenstein, *Philosophical Investigations*: §293).
21. Stanley Cavell, "In Quest of the Ordinary: Texts of Recovery," in *Romanticism and Contemporary Criticism*, ed. M. Eaves and M. Fischer (Cornell University Press, 1986): 184.
22. Stanley Cavell, "Knowing and Acknowledging," in *Must We Mean What We Say?* (Cambridge University Press, 1976): 246–247 (hereafter *Acknow.*).
23. Stanley Cavell, "In Quest of the Ordinary": 184.
24. Adam Smith, *The Theory of Moral Sentiments* (Cambridge University Press, 2002): 12. See also Martha Nussbaum's remarks on Smith in *Upheavals of Thought: The Intelligence of Emotions* (Cambridge University Press, 2003): 309–310.
25. With this, Cavell interestingly converges with Levinas. On the relationship between Wittgenstein, Cavell, and Levinas, see Hent De Vries, "From 'Ghost in the Machine' to 'Spiritual Automaton': Philosophical Meditation in Wittgenstein, Cavell and Levinas," *International Journal of the Philosophy of Religion* 60 (2006): 77–97.

26. Stanley Cavell, *In Quest of the Ordinary: Lines of Skepticism and Romanticism* (University of Chicago Press, 1988): 187.
27. Ludwig Wittgenstein, *On Certainty*, ed. G. E. M. Anscombe and G. H. Wright (Harper Torch Books, 1972): 49 (§378).
28. Stephen Mulhall, *Stanley Cavell: Philosophy's Recounting of the Ordinary* (Oxford University Press, 1994): 110. For an illuminating account of Cavell and the problem of skepticism, see pp. 94–114 of Mulhall's book. See also David Macarthur, "Cavell on Skepticism and the Importance of Not-Knowing," *Conversations: Journal of Cavellian Studies* 2 (2014): 2–23.
29. Stanley Cavell, *The Claim of Reason*: 84.
30. Veena Das, "Language and Body: Transactions in the Construction of Pain," *Daedalus* 125, no. 1 (1996): 88.
31. See Edward Mooney, "Acknowledgement, Suffering, and Praise: Stanley Cavell as Religious Continental Thinker," *Soundings: An Interdisciplinary Journal* 88, no. 3–4 (2005): 393–411.
32. See Emmanuel Levinas, *Entre nous: On Thinking-of-the-Other*, trans. Michael B. Smith (Columbia University Press, 1998) and especially, "Useless Suffering," in ibid.: 91–101.
33. Knox, *The Heroic Temper*: 132.
34. Richard T. Eldridge, "Introduction: Between Acknowledgement and Avoidance," in *Stanley Cavell*, ed. Richard T. Eldridge (Cambridge University Press, 2003): 1; Cf. Richard T. Eldridge and Bernard Rhie, eds., *Stanley Cavell and Literary Studies: Consequences of Skepticism* (Continuum, 2011): esp. 106–119, and Richard T. Eldridge, "Philosophy and the Achievement of Community: Rorty, Cavell, and Criticism," *Metaphilosophy* 14 (1983): 107–125.
35. Hall points out the difference between Neoptolemus' response, which she characterizes as the "sympathetic, non-intrusive, listening presence of another human being," and the chorus, which seems at first to be sympathetic toward Philoctetes' suffering, a sympathy that gradually proves to be qualified. The chorus represents the position of a community that offers help to Philoctetes, yet as soon as he denies, turns its back to him. See Hall, "Ancient Greek Responses to Suffering": 164–165.
36. Mulhall, *Stanley Cavell*: 139–140.
37. I thank Eli Friedlander for our conversations about Cavell and this issue in particular.
38. For an interesting discussion of touch in Sophocles' *Philoctetes*, see Jennifer Clarke Kosak, "Therapeutic Touch and Sophokles' *Philoktetes*," *Harvard Studies in Classical Philology* 99 (1999): 93–134.
39. My use of the term draws from Werner Hamacher's "Afformative, Strike," trans. Dana Hollander, *Cardozo Law Review* 13, no. 4 (1991): 1133–1157 (hereafter *AF*).
40. André Gide, *Philoctetes; or, the Treatise on Three Ethics*, trans. Oscar Mandel, in *Philoctetes and the Fall of Troy: Documents, Iconography, Interpretations*, ed. Oscar Mandel (University of Nebraska Press, 1981): 162–178 (hereafter *Gide, Philoc.*).
41. Earlier in the play, when he is alone on the stage, Philoctetes laments Ulysses' cold heartedness, his betrayal, and his cunning. He contemplates using his bow against him, when a sound of approaching footsteps is heard. Philoctetes seizes his bow but then sees Neoptolemus and puts it down. Though Neoptolemus was part of the scheme, he has listened to Philoctetes and eventually asked him to teach him virtue. This saves his life (*Gide, Philoc.* 172).
42. See also Heidegger's discussion of Knut Hamsun's "The Road Leads On" (which belongs together with his "The Wayfarer" and "August"). Heidegger describes the figure of August "who embodies the uprooted, universal know-how of today's humanity, but in the form of a Dasein that cannot lose its ties to the unfamiliar, because in its despairing powerlessness it remains genuine and superior. In his last days, this August is alone in the high mountains. The poet says: 'He sits here between his ears and hears true emptiness. Quite amusing, a fancy. On the ocean (earlier, August often went to sea) something stirred (at least), and there, there was a sound, something audible, a water chorus. Here—nothing meets nothing and is not there, there is not even a hole. One can only shake one's head in resignation.' " (*Introduction to Metaphysics*, trans. Gregory Fried and Richard Plot [Yale University Press, 2000]: 28–29 [20–21]). August represents something of Heidegger's idea of the relationship between scientific (communicative, referential) language and the language and nothingness that can only be expressed by the philosopher and the poet: "One cannot, in fact, talk about and deal with Nothing as if it were a thing, such as the rain out there, or a mountain, or any object at

all; Nothing remains in principle inaccessible to all science. Whoever truly wants to talk of Nothing must necessarily become unscientific. . . . [T]he poet always speaks as if beings were expressed and addressed for the first time. In the poetry of the poet and in the thinking of the thinker, there is always so much world-space to spare that each and every thing—a tree, a mountain, a house, the call of a bird—completely loses its indifference and familiarity. True talk of Nothing always remains unfamiliar. It does not allow itself to be made common. It dissolves, to be sure, if one places it in the cheap acid of a merely logical cleverness. This is why we cannot begin to speak about Nothing immediately, as we can in describing a picture, for example. But the possibility of such speech about Nothing can be indicated" (*IM* 27-28 [19–20]). I thank Werner Hamacher for pointing out these passages to me.

43. Wilson, "Philoctetes: The Wound and the Bow": 289.
44. An interesting echo of this structure can be found in the story of Telephus who was wounded in his hip by Achilles' spear, a wound that could only be cured by what caused it. A kind of homeopathic (or sympathetic) principle is at work here. The wound allows for healing: in the case of Philoctetes, his disintegrated language is also the key for its reemergence. The story of Telephus was told in many versions, including those of Sophocles, *Fragments*, ed. and trans. Hugh Lloyd-Jones, Loeb Classical Library 483 (Harvard University Press, 1996): 290–299) and Euripides, *Fragments: Oedipus-Chrysippus. Other Fragments*, ed. and trans. Christopher Collard and Martin Cropp (Harvard University Press, 2009): 195–223.
45. I have also developed this argument in the context of Gershom Scholem's early writings on the linguistic structure of lament; see Ilit Ferber, "A Language of the Border: On Scholem's Theory of Lament," *Journal of Jewish Thought and Philosophy* 12, no. 2 (2013): 161–186.
46. A previous version of the following pages was published in Ilit Ferber, "Wandering about Language," *Philosophy Today* 61, no. 4 (2017): 1005–1012.
47. Werner Hamacher, "Other Pains," trans. Ian Alexander Moore, *Philosophy Today* 61, no. 4 (2017): 965 (hereafter *Pains*).
48. Werner Hamacher, "95 Theses on Philology," trans. Catherine Diehl, *Diacritis* 39, no. 1 (2009): 25–44 (hereafter *Theses*).
49. Personal correspondence, June 3, 2014.
50. Werner Hamacher, "The Second Inversion: Movements of a Figure through Celan's Poetry," in *Premises: Essays on Philosophy and Literature from Kant to Celan*, trans. Peter Fenves (Harvard University Press, 1996): 337. See also Daniel Heller-Roazen, "Language, or No Language," *Diacritics* 29, no. 3: 22–39.
51. It belongs in this sense to a line of authors such as Benjamin, Heidegger, and Derrida, who similarly questioned, criticized, and wrestled with these conceptions. See, for instance, Derrida's description of Hamacher's text as "impressive, admirable and original," adding: "There is, despite appearances, nothing paradoxical about the fact that I say very little about his essay here, contenting myself with inviting the reader to read and reread it while weighing its every word" (Jacques Derrida, "Marx & Sons," in *Ghostly Demarcations: A Symposium on Jacques Derrida's Specters of Marx*, ed. Michael Sprinker [London: Verso, 1999]: 224–225).
52. Hamacher, "The Second Inversion": 355.
53. Hamacher, *AF*: 1133–1157.
54. Werner Hamacher, "The Promise of Interpretation," *Premises*: 128–129, quoted by Daniel Heller-Roazen, "Language, or No Language," *Diacritics* 29, no. 3 (1999): 31.

Chapter 6

1. I elaborate on these two paradigms in chapter 1.
2. Aristotle, *De Interpretatione*: chapters 4–6. It is interesting to note that Aristotle ends his short discussion of linguistic propositions with a remark on prayer, which he understands as a linguistic form that does not obey the above explanation and is "neither true or false" (17a 1–4).
3. Hamacher, "The Second Inversion": 338.
4. J. L. Austin, *How to Do Things with Words* (Oxford University Press, 1962): 1. The text is based on a series of lectures Austin gave at Harvard University in 1955.
5. Austin, *How to Do Things with Words*: 8. See also Shoshana Felman's discussion of Austin's use of the terms "felicity" and "infelicity" (i.e., for success and failure) in reference to performative

language in her *The Scandal of the Speaking Body: Don Juan with J. L. Austin, or Seduction in Two Languages* (Stanford University Press, 1980): 7.

6. Hagi Kenaan, "Language, Philosophy and the Risk of Failure: Rereading the Debate between Searle and Derrida," *Continental Philosophy Review* 35 (2002): 117–133. Kenaan not only provides a detailed account of the problematic implications of Austin's theory but also elaborates on Searle's and Derrida's position vis-à-vis Austin's. Although he does not mention pain or any other extreme sensation, Kenaan's argument is important to my own discussion as it focus on "successful" language and what it leaves out of the discussion, or for that matter, out of sight.
7. I present an elaborate version of these claims in "Language Failing: The Reach of Lament," talk given at the ICI (Institute for Cultural Inquiry, Berlin) on May 11, 2015.
8. Personal correspondence, June 3, 2014. See also my discussion in chapter 6.
9. Werner Hamacher, "The Promise of Interpretation," in *Premises*: 128–129, quoted by Daniel Heller-Roazen, "Language, or No Language," *Diacritics* 29, no.3 (1999): 31.

BIBLIOGRAPHY

Agamben, Giorgio. *Infancy and History: On the Destruction of Experience*, trans. Liz Heron. Verso, 2007.

Agamben, Giorgio. *Language and Death: The Place of Negativity*. University of Minnesota Press, 2006.

Agamben, Giorgio. *The Open: Man and Animal*, trans. Kevin Attell. Stanford University Press, 2004.

Agamben, Giorgio. *Remnants of Auschwitz*, trans. Daniel Heller-Roazen. Zone Books, 1999.

Améry, Jean. *At the Mind's Limits: Contemplations by a Survivor on Auschwitz and Its Realities*, trans. Sidney Rosenfeld and Stella P. Rosenfeld. Indiana University Press, 1980.

Arendt, Hannah. *The Human Condition*. University of Chicago Press, 1998.

Asad, Talal. *Formations of the Secular: Christianity, Islam, Modernity*. Stanford University Press, 2003.

Austin, J. L. *How to Do Things with Words*. Oxford University Press, 1962.

Barnard, F. M. *Herder's Social and Political Thought from Enlightenment to Nationalism*. Clarendon Press, 1967.

Bataille, Georges. *Inner Experience*, trans. Leslie Anne Boldt. State University of New York Press, 1988.

Bauman, Thomas. *North German Opera in the Age of Goethe*. Cambridge University Press, 1985.

Beiser, Frederick C. "Berlin and the German Counter-Enlightenment." In *Isaiah Berlin's Counter-Enlightenment*, ed. Joseph Mali and Robert Wokler. *Transactions of the American Philosophical Society* 93, no. 5 (2003): 105–116.

Beiser, Frederick C. *The Fate of Reason: German Philosophy from Kant to Fichte*. Harvard University Press, 1987.

Bending, Lucy. *The Representation of Bodily Pain in Late Nineteenth-Century English Culture*. Oxford University Press, 2000.

Benjamin, Walter. "Outline of the Psychophysical Problem." In *Selected Writings*, vol. 1 (1913–1926), trans. Rodney Livingstone, ed. Marcus Bullock and Michael W. Jennings, 393–401. Harvard University Press, 1996.

Berlin, Isaiah. *Vico and Herder: Two Studies in the History of Ideas*. Chatto & Windus, 1976.

Blanchot, Maurice. *The Infinite Conversation*, trans. Susan Hanson. University of Minnesota Press, 2003.

Blanchot, Maurice. *The Unavowable Community*. Station Hill Press, 1988.

Blok, Vincent. "An Indication of Being—Reflections on Heidegger's Engagement with Ernst Jünger." *Journal of the British Society for Phenomenology* 42, no. 2 (2011): 194–208.

Brogan, Walter. "Listening to the Silence: Reticence and the Call of Conscience in Heidegger's Philosophy." In *Heidegger and Language*, ed. Jeffrey Powel, 32–45. Indiana University Press, 2013.

Bruns, Gerald L. "Language, Pain and Fear." *Iowa Review* 11, no. 2/3 (1980).

Budelmann, Felix. "The Reception of Sophocles' Representation of Physical Pain." *American Journal of Philology* 128, no. 4 (2007): 443–467.

Cassirer, Ernest. *The Philosophy of Symbolic Forms*, vol. 1. Yale University Press, 1966.

Cassirer, Ernst. *The Problem of Knowledge: Philosophy, Science and History since Hegel*, trans. William H. Woglom and Charles W. Hendel. Yale University Press, 1950.

Cavell, Stanley. *The Claim of Reason: Wittgenstein, Skepticism, Morality, and Tragedy*. Oxford University Press, 1999.

Cavell, Stanley. "Comments on Veena Das's Essay 'Language and Body: Transactions in the Construction of Pain.'" *Daedalus* 125, no. 1 (1996).

Cavell, Stanley. *In Quest of the Ordinary: Lines of Skepticism and Romanticism*. University of Chicago Press, 1988.

Cavell, Stanley. "In Quest of the Ordinary: Texts of Recovery." In *Romanticism and Contemporary Criticism*, ed. M. Eaves and M. Fischer, 183-213. Cornell University Press, 1986.

Cavell, Stanley. "Knowing and Acknowledging." In *Must We Mean What We Say?*, 238–266. Cambridge University Press, 1976.

Cioran, Emil M. *On the Heights of Despair*, trans. Ilinca Zarifopol-Johnston. University of Chicago Press, 1992.

Comay, Rebecca. "Paradoxes of Lament: Benjamin and Hamlet." In *Lament in Jewish Thought: Philosophical, Theological, and Literary Perspectives*, ed. Ilit Ferber and Paula Schwebel, 257–275. De Gruyter, 2014.

Cover, Robert M. "Violence and the Word." *Yale Faculty Scholarship Series*, paper 2708 (1986): 1601–1629.

Dahlstrom, Daniel O. "The Aesthetic Holism of Hamann, Herder and Schiller." In *The Cambridge Companion to German Idealism*, ed. Karl Ameriks, 76–94. Cambridge University Press, 2017.

Das, Veena. "Language and Body: Transactions in the Construction of Pain." *Daedalus* 125, no. 1 (1996): 67–91.

Daudet, Alphonse. *In the Land of Pain*, trans. Julian Barnes. Knopf, 2003.

De la Durantaye, Leland. *Giorgio Agamben: A Critical Introduction*. Stanford University Press, 2009.

De Man, Paul. *Allegories of Reading: Figural Language in Rousseau, Nietzsche, Rilke, and Proust*. Yale University Press, 1979.

De Man, Paul. "The Rhetoric of Blindness: Jacques Derrida's Reading of Rousseau." In *Blindness and Insight: Essays in the Rhetoric of Contemporary Criticism*, 102–141. Oxford University Press, 1971.

Derrida, Jacques. "Heidegger's Ear." In *Remembering Heidegger: Commemorations*, ed. John Sallis, 163–218. Indiana University Press, 1993.

Derrida, Jacques. "Marx & Sons." In *Ghostly Demarcations: A Symposium on Jacques Derrida's Specters of Marx*, ed. Michael Sprinker, 213–269. London: Verso, 1999.

Derrida, Jacques. *Of Grammatology*, trans. G. C. Spivak. Johns Hopkins University Press, 1997.

DeSouza, Nigel. "Language, Reason, and Sociability: Herder's Critique of Rousseau." *Intellectual History Review* 22, no. 2 (2012): 221–240.

De Vries, Hent. "From 'Ghost in the Machine' to 'Spiritual Automaton': Philosophical Meditation in Wittgenstein, Cavell and Levinas." *International Journal of the Philosophy of Religion* 60 (2006): 77–97.

Dickinson, Emily. *The Complete Poems of Emily Dickinson*, ed. Thomas H. Johnson, poem 650. Little, Brown, 1960.

Dugdale, Eric. "Philoctetes." In *Brill's Companion to the Reception of Sophocles*, ed. R. Lauriola and K. N. Demetriou, 77–145. Brill, 2017.

Eldridge, Richard T. "Introduction: Between Acknowledgement and Avoidance." In *Stanley Cavell*, ed. Richard T. Eldridge, 1–14. Cambridge University Press, 2003.

Eldridge, Richard T. "Philosophy and the Achievement of Community: Rorty, Cavell, and Criticism." *Metaphilosophy* 14 (1983): 107–125.

Eldridge, Richard T., and Bernard Rhie, eds. *Stanley Cavell and Literary Studies: Consequences of Skepticism*. Continuum, 2011.

Euripides. *Fragments: Oedipus-Chrysippus. Other Fragments*, ed. and trans. Christopher Collard and Martin Cropp. Harvard University Press, 2009.

Felman, Shoshana. *The Scandal of the Speaking Body: Don Juan with J. L. Austin, or Seduction in Two Languages*. Stanford University Press, 1980.

Fenves, Peter. *Late Kant: Towards Another Law of the Earth*. Routledge, 2003.

Ferber, Ilit. "Aphasie, Trauma und Freuds schmerzlose Wunde." In *Freuds Referenzen*, ed. C. Kirchhoff and G. Scharbert, 145–167. Kulturverlag Kadmos Berlin, 2012.

Ferber, Ilit. "A Language of the Border: On Scholem's Theory of Lament." *Journal of Jewish Thought and Philosophy* 12, no. 2 (2013): 161–186.

Ferber, Ilit. "Pain as Yardstick: Jean Améry." *Journal of French and Francophone Philosophy* 24, no. 3 (2016): 3–16.

Ferber, Ilit. "'Schmerz war ein Staudamm': Benjamin on Pain." *Benjamin-Studien* 3 (2014): 165–177.

Ferber, Ilit. "Wandering about Language." *Philosophy Today* 61, no. 4 (2017): 1005–1012.

Ferber, Ilit. "A Wound without Pain: Freud on Aphasia." *Naharaim: Journal of German Jewish Literature and Cultural History* 4 (2010): 133–151.

Fitzpatrick, Peter. "Why the Law Is also Nonviolent." In *Law, Violence, and the Possibility of Justice*, ed. Austin Sarat, 142–173. Princeton University Press, 2001.

Forrester, John. *Language and the Origins of Psychoanalysis*. Macmillan, 1980.

Forster, Michael N. "Gods, Animals, and Artists: Some Problem Cases in Herder's Philosophy of Language." *Inquiry* 46, no. 1 (2003): 65–96.

Forster, Michael N. "Herder's Philosophy of Language, Interpretation, and Translation: Three Fundamental Principles." *Review of Metaphysics* 56, no. 2 (2002): 323–356.

Freud, Sigmund. *Extracts from the Fliess Papers* ("Draft G: Melancholia"). *The Standard Edition of the Complete Psychological Works of Sigmund Freud*, vol. 1 (1886–1899), ed. James Strachey, 200–206. Hogarth Press and the Institute of Psycho-analysis, 1959.

Freud, Sigmund. "Inhibitions, Symptoms, Anxiety." *The Standard Edition of the Complete Psychological Works of Sigmund Freud*, vol. 20 (1925–1926), ed. James Strachey, 75–176. Hogarth Press and the Institute of Psycho-analysis, 1959.

Freud, Sigmund. "Mourning and Melancholia." *The Standard Edition of the Complete Psychological Works of Sigmund Freud*, vol. 4 (1914–1916), ed. James Strachey, 243–258. Hogarth Press and the Institute of Psycho-analysis, 1959.

Freud, Sigmund. "On Narcissism: An Introduction." *The Standard Edition of the Complete Psychological Works of Sigmund Freud*, vol. 14 (1914–1916), ed. James Strachey, 67–102. Hogarth Press and the Institute of Psycho-analysis, 1959.

Friedlander, Eli. *J. J. Rousseau: An Afterlife of Words*. Harvard University Press, 2004.

Gide, André. *Philoctetes; or, the Treatise on Three Ethics*, trans. Oscar Mandel. In *Philoctetes and the Fall of Troy: Documents, Iconography, Interpretations*, ed. Oscar Mandel, 158–178. University of Nebraska Press, 1981.

Greenberg, Valerie D. *Freud and His Aphasia Book*. Cornell University Press, 1997.

Gustafson, Susan E. and McCormick. "Sadomasochism, Mutilation, and Men: Lessing's 'Laokoon,' Herder's 'Kritische Wälder,' Gerstenberg's 'Ugolino,' and the Storm and Stress of Drama." *Poetics Today* 20, no. 2 ("Lessing's Laokoon: Context and Reception") (1999): 197–218.

Hall, Edith. "Ancient Greek Responses to Suffering: Thinking with Philoctetes." In *Perspectives on Human Suffering*, ed. J. Malpas and N. Lickiss, 155–169. Springer, 2012.

Hamacher Werner. "Afformative, Strike," trans. Dana Hollander. *Cardozo Law Review* 13, no. 4 (1991): 1133–1157.

Hamacher, Werner. "95 Theses on Philology," trans. Catherine Diehl. *Diacritis* 39, no. 1 (2009): 25–44.

Hamacher, Werner. "Other Pains," trans. Ian Alexander Moore. *Philosophy Today* 61, no. 4 (2017): 963–989.

Hamacher, Werner. "The Promise of Interpretation." In *Premises: Essays on Philosophy and Literature from Kant to Celan*, trans. Peter Fenves, 81–142. Harvard University Press, 1996.

Hamacher, Werner. "The Second Inversion: Movements of a Figure through Celan's Poetry." In *Premises: Essays on Philosophy and Literature from Kant to Celan*, trans. Peter Fenves, 337–387. Harvard University Press, 1996.

Hamann, Johann Georg. *Writings on Philosophy and Language*, ed. and trans. Kenneth Haynes. Cambridge University Press, 2007.

Hanly, Peter. "Dark Celebration: Heidegger's Silent Music." In *Heidegger and Language*, ed. Jeffrey Powel. Indiana University Press, 2013.

Hanly, Peter. "Marking Silence: Heidegger and Herder on Word and Origin." *Studies in Christian Philosophy* (*Studia Philosophiae Christianae*) 4 (2013): 69–86.

Heaney, Seamus. *The Cure at Troy: A Version of Sophocles' Philoctetes*. Farrar, Straus and Giroux, 1991.

Hegel, Georg Wilhelm Friedrich. *Hegel's Philosophy of Subjective Spirit*, vol. 2, *Anthropology*, trans. and ed. M. J. Petry. D. Reidel, 1978.

Heidegger, Martin. *Being and Time*, trans. Joan Stambaugh. State University of New York Press, 1992.

Heidegger, Martin. *Bremen and Freiburg Lectures: Insight into That Which Is and Basic Principles of Thinking*, trans. Andrew J. Mitchell. Indiana University Press, 2012.

Heidegger, Martin. *Contributions to Philosophy (From Enowning)*, trans. Parvis Emad and Kenneth Maly. Indiana University Press, 1999.

Heidegger, Martin. *The Event*, trans. Richard Rojcewicz. Indiana University Press, 2013.

Heidegger, Martin. *The Fundamental Concepts of Metaphysics: World, Finitude, Solitude*, trans. William Mc Neill and Nicolas Walker. Indiana University Press, 1955.

Heidegger, Martin. *Gesamtausgabe*, ed. Ingrid Schüßler. Vittorio Klostermann GmbH, 1999.

Heidegger, Martin. *History of the Concept of Time: Prolegomena*, trans. Theodore Kisiel. Indiana University Press, 1985.

Heidegger, Martin. *Introduction to Metaphysics*, trans. Gregory Fried and Richard Polt. Yale University Press, 2000.

Heidegger, Martin. "Language." In *Poetry, Language, Thought*, trans. Albert Hofstadter, 185–208. Harper Perennial, 2001.

Heidegger, Martin. "Letter on 'Humanism.'" In *Pathmarks*, ed. William McNeill, trans. Frank A. Capuzzi, 239–276. Cambridge University Press, 1998.

Heidegger, Martin. "Logos (Heraclitus, Fragment B 50)." In *Early Greek Thinking: The Dawn of Western Philosophy*, trans. David Farrell Krell and Frank A. Capuzzi, 59–78. Harper & Row, 1984.

Heidegger, Martin. *Nietzsche: Volumes I and II*, trans. David Farrell Krell. Harper & Row, 1979.

Heidegger, Martin. *On the Essence of Language: The Metaphysics of Language and the Essencing of the Word. Concerning Herder's Treatise on the Origin of Language*, trans. Wanda Torres Gregory and Yvonna Unna. State University of New York Press, 2004.

Heidegger, Martin, "On the Question of Being." In *Pathmarks*, trans. William McNeill, 291–322. Cambridge University Press, 1998.

Heidegger, Martin. *Vom Wesen der Sprache: Die Metaphysik der Sprache und die Wesung des Wortes. Zu Herders Abhandlung "Über den Ursprung der Sprache"*. In *Gesamtausgabe*, vol. 85, ed. Ingrid Schüßler. Vittorio Klostermann GmbH, 1999.

Heidegger, Martin. "What Are Poets For?" In *Poetry, Language, Thought*, trans. Albert Hofstadter, 87–139. Harper Perennial, 2001.

Heidegger, Martin, and Eugen Fink. *Heraclitus Seminar 1966/67*, trans. Charles H. Seibert. University of Alabama Press, 1979.

Heller-Roazen, Daniel. "Language, or No Language." *Diacritics* 29, no. 3 (1999): 22–39.

Herder, Johann Gottfried. *Abhandlung über den Ursprung der Sprache*. In *Werke*: Bd. 1: Frühe Schriften 1764–1772, ed. Urich Gaier, 697–810. Deutscher Klassiker Verlag, 1985.

Herder, Johann Gottfried. "First Grove, Dedicated to Mr. Lessing's Laocoön." In *Selected Writings on Aesthetics*, ed. and trans. Gregory Moore, 51–176. Princeton University Press, 2006.

Herder, Johann Gottfried. "Fourth Grove, On Riedel's Theory of the Beaux Arts." In *Selected Writings on Aesthetics*, ed. and trans. Gregory Moore, 177–290. Princeton University Press, 2006.

Herder, Johann Gottfried. "Fragments on Recent German Literature." In *Philosophical Writings*, trans. and ed. Michael N. Forster, 33–64. Cambridge University Press, 2002.

Herder, Johann Gottfried. "Kritische Wälder oder Betrachtungen, die Wissenschaft und Kunst des Schönen betreffend." In *Schriften zur Ästhetik und Literatur, 1767–1781*, vol. 2 of Johann Gottfried Herder, *Werke*, ed. Günter E. Grimm, 57–245. Deutscher Klassiker Verlag, 1993.

Herder, Johann Gottfried. "On Cognition and Sensation of the Human Soul." In *Philosophical Writings*, trans. and ed. Michael N. Forster, 187–243. Cambridge University Press, 2002.

Herder, Johann Gottfried. *Outlines of a Philosophy of the History of Man*, trans. T. Churchill. Bergman, 1800; republished in 2016 by Random Shack.

Herder, Johann Gottfried. "Philoktetes: Szenen mit Gesang." In *Nachlaß veröffentlicht, Sämmtliche Werke*. [Abt.] Zur schönen Literatur und Kunst 6. Theil, ed. J. G. Herder, 113–126. Cotta, 1806.

Herder, Johann Gottfried. *Sculpture: Some Observations on Shape and Form from Pygmalion's Creative Dream*, trans. Jason Gaiger. University of Chicago Press, 2002.

Herder, Johann Gottfried. *Selected Writings on Aesthetics*, ed. and trans. Gregory Moore. Princeton University Press, 2006.

Herder, Johann Gottfried. "Treatise on the Origin of Language." In *Philosophical Writings*, trans. and ed. Michael N. Forster, 65–164. Cambridge University Press, 2002.

Hume, David. *A Treatise of Human Nature*, ed. D. F. Norton and M. J. Norton. Oxford University Press, 2000.

Hyslop, Alec. *Other Minds*. Kluwer, 1995.

Inwood, Michael. *A Heidegger Dictionary*. Blackwell, 1999.

Kant, Immanuel. *Anthropology, History, and Education*, ed. and trans. Robert B. Louden. Cambridge University Press, 2007.

Kenaan, Hagi. "Language, Philosophy and the Risk of Failure: Rereading the Debate Between Searle and Derrida." *Continental Philosophy Review* 35 (2002): 117–133.

Kenaan, Hagi. *The Present Personal: Philosophy and the Hidden Face of Language*. Columbia University Press, 2005.

Kittler, Friedrich. *Discourse Networks 1800/1900*, trans. Michael Metteer with Chris Cullens. Stanford University Press, 1990.

Knox, Bernard M. W. *The Heroic Temper: Studies in Sophoclean Tragedy*. University of California Press, 1983.

Kosak, Jennifer Clarke. "Therapeutic Touch and Sophokles' *Philoktetes*." *Harvard Studies in Classical Philology* 99 (1999): 93–134.

Kovacs, George. "Heidegger in Dialogue with Herder: Crossing the Language of Metaphysics toward Be-ing-historical Language." *Heidegger Studies* 17 (2001): 45–63.

Lessing, Gotthold Ephraim. *Laocoön: An Essay on the Limits of Painting and Poetry*, trans. Edward Allen McCormick. Johns Hopkins University Press, 1962.

Lestition, Steven. "Countering, Transposing, or Negating the Enlightenment? A Response to Robert Norton." *Journal of the History of Ideas* 6, no. 4 (2007): 659–681.

Levinas, Emmanuel. *Entre Nous: On Thinking-of-the-Other*, trans. Michael B. Smith and Barbara Harshav. Columbia University Press, 1998.

Levinas, Emmanuel. *Time and the Other*, trans. Richard Cohen. Duquesne University Press, 1987.

Levinas, Emmanuel. "Useless Suffering." In *Entre nous: On Thinking-of-the-Other*, trans. Michael B. Smith and Barbara Harshav. Columbia University Press, 1998.

Lewis, C. S. *The Problem of Pain*. Harper Collins, 2015.

Lifschitz, Avi. *Language and the Enlightenment: The Berlin Debates of the Eighteenth Century*. Oxford University Press, 2012.

Lifschitz, Avi. "Language as a Means and an Obstacle to Freedom: The Case of Moses Mendelssohn." In *Freedom and the Construction of Europe*, vol. 2, ed. Quentin Skinner and Martin van Gelderen, 84–102. Cambridge University Press, 2013.

Macarthur, David. "Cavell on Skepticism and the Importance of Not-Knowing." *Conversations: Journal of Cavellian Studies* 2 (2014): 2–23.

Mandel, Oscar, ed. *Philoctetes and the Fall of Troy: Documents, Iconography, Interpretations*. University of Nebraska Press, 1981.

Marion, Jean-Luc. *In Excess: Studies of Saturated Phenomena*, trans. Robyn Horner and Vincent Berraud. Fordham University Press, 2002.

Marshall, David. *The Figure of Theater: Shaftesbury, Defoe, Adam Smith, and George Eliot*. Columbia University Press, 1986.

Marshall, David. *The Surprising Effects of Sympathy: Marivaux, Diderot, Rousseau, and Mary Shelley*. Chicago University Press, 1988.

Mendelssohn, Moses. "Sendschreiben an den Herrn Magister Lessing in Leipzig." In *Gesammelte Schriften Jubiläumsausgabe*, vol. 2, ed. F. Bamberger et al., 81–110. Friedrich Fromman Verlag, 1972.

Meyer, Matthew. "Reflective Listening in Heraclitus." *International Journal of Listening* 21, no. 1 (2007): 57–65.

Mitchell, Andrew J. "Entering the World of Pain: Heidegger." *Telos* 150 (2010): 83–96.

Mitchell, W. J. T. "The Politics of Genre: Space and Time in Lessing's Laocoon." *Representations* 6 (1984): 98–115.

Mooney, Edward. "Acknowledgement, Suffering, and Praise: Stanley Cavell as Religious Continental Thinker." *Soundings: An Interdisciplinary Journal* 88, no. 3–4 (2005): 393–411.

Moore, Gregory. "Introduction." In Herder, Johann Gottfried, *Selected Writings on Aesthetics*, trans. and ed. Gregory Moore. Princeton University Press, 2006.

Morris, David B. *The Culture of Pain*. University of California Press, 1993.

von Mücke, Dorothea E. *Virtue and the Veil of Illusion: Generic Innovation and the Pedagogical Project in Eighteenth-Century Literature*. Stanford University Press, 1991.

Mulhall, Stephen. *Stanley Cavell: Philosophy's Recounting of the Ordinary*. Oxford University Press, 1994.

Müller, Heiner. "Philoctetes." In *Philoctetes and the Fall of Troy*, trans. Oscar Mandel in collaboration with Maria Kelsen Feder, 222–250. University of Nebraska Press, 1981.

Nagel, Thomas. *The View from Nowhere*. Oxford University Press, 1986.

Nancy, Jean-Luc. *The Inoperative Community*. University of Minnesota Press, 1991.

Norton, Robert. "Isaiah Berlin's 'Expressionism,' or: 'Ha! Du Bist das Blökende!'" *Journal of the History of Ideas* 69, no. 2 (2008): 339–347.

Norton, Robert E. "The Myth of the Counter-Enlightenment." *Journal of the History of Ideas* 68, no. 4 (2007): 635–658.

Nussbaum, Martha. *Upheavals of Thought: The Intelligence of Emotions*. Cambridge University Press, 2003.

Oliver, Kelly. *Animal Lessons: How They Teach Us to Be Human*. Columbia University Press, 2009.

Pontalis, J.-B. "On Psychic Pain." In *Frontiers in Psychoanalysis: Between the Dream and Psychic Pain*, trans. Catherine Cullen and Philip Cullen, 149–205. International Universities Press, 1981.

Proß, Wolfgang. *Johann Gottfried Herder, Abhandlung über den Ursprung der Sprache: Text, Materialen, Kommentar*. Carl Hanser Verlag, 1978.

Ricoeur, Paul. "Violence and Language." In *Political and Social Essays*, 32–41. Ohio University Press, 1974.

Rilke, Rainer Maria. *Sonnets to Orpheus*, trans. Willis Barnstone. Shambhala, 2004.

Rizzuto, Anna-Maria. "Freud's Speech Apparatus and Spontaneous Speech." *International Journal of Psycho-Analysis* 74 (1993): 113–127.

Rousseau, Jean-Jacques. "Discourse on the Origin and Foundations of Inequality among Men *or* Second Discourse." In *The Discourses and Other Early Political Writings*, trans. and ed. Victor Gourevitch, 111–188. Cambridge University Press, 1997.

Rousseau, Jean-Jacques. *Emile or on Education*, trans. Alan Bloom. Basic Books, 1979.

Rousseau, Jean-Jacques. "The Essay on the Origin of Languages in Which Melody and Musical Imitation Are Treated." In *The Discourses and Other Early Political Writings*, trans. and ed. Victor Gourevitch, 247–299. Cambridge University Press, 1997.

Rousseau, Jean-Jacques. "Examination of Two Principles Advanced by M. Rameau in His Brochure Entitled: 'Errors on Music in the Encyclopedia.'" In *Essay on the Origin of Languages and Writings Related to Music* (*Collected Writings of Rousseau,* vol. 7), trans. and ed. John T. Scott, 271–288. University Press of New England, 1998.

Rudowski, Victor Anthony. "Lessing Contra Winckelmann." *Journal of Aesthetics and Art Criticism* 44, no. 3 (1986): 235–243.

Scarry, Elaine. *The Body in Pain: The Making and Unmaking of the World.* Oxford University Press, 1985.

Sikka, Sonia. "Heidegger's Concept of Volk." *Philosophical Forum* 26, no. 2 (1994): 101–126.

Sikka, Sonia. "Herder's Critique of Pure Reason." *Review of Metaphysics* 61, no. 1 (2007): 31–50.

Sikka, Sonia. *Herder on Humanity and Cultural Difference: Enlightened Relativism.* Cambridge University Press, 2011.

Sikka, Sonia. "Herder on the Relation between Language and World." *History of Philosophy Quarterly* 21, no. 2 (2004): 183–200.

Singer, Peter. "Unspeakable Acts" (review of E. Scarry, *The Body in Pain: The Making and Unmaking of the World* and E. Peters, *Torture*). *New York Review of Books,* February 27, 1986.

Smith, Adam. *The Theory of Moral Sentiment,* ed. Knud Haakonssen. Cambridge University Press, 2002.

Smith, Peter, and O. R. Jones. *The Philosophy of Mind: An Introduction.* Cambridge University Press, 1986.

Sontag, Susan. *Illness as Metaphor.* Farrar, Straus and Giroux, 1978.

Sophocles. *Fragments,* ed. and trans. Hugh Lloyd-Jones. Loeb Classical Library 483. Harvard University Press, 1996.

Sophocles. "Philoctetes." In *Antigone, The Women of Trachis, Philoctetes, Oedipus at Colonus,* ed. and trans. Hugh Lloyd-Jones. Loeb Classical Library 21. Harvard University Press, 1998.

Sophocles. "Philoctetes." In *Four Tragedies, Ajax, Women of Trachis, Electra, Philoctetes.* trans. Peter Meineck and Paul Woodruff. Hacket Publishing, 2007.

Stephens, J. Ceri. "The Wound of Philoctetes." *Mnemosyne* 48 (1995): 153–168.

Taylor, Charles. *Hegel.* Cambridge University Press, 1975.

Taylor, Charles. "Heidegger, Language, and Ecology." In *Philosophical Arguments,* 100–126. Harvard University Press, 1995.

Taylor, Charles. "The Importance of Herder." In *Isaiah Berlin: A Celebration,* ed. Edna and Ullmann-Margalit and Avishai Margalit, 40–63. University of Chicago Press, 1991.

Taylor, Charles. *The Language Animal: The Full Shape of the Human Linguistic Capacity.* Harvard University Press, 2016.

Taylor, Charles. *Sources of the Self: The Making of the Modern Identity.* Cambridge University Press, 1989.

Terada, Rei. *Feeling in Theory: Emotion after the "Death of the Subject."* Harvard University Press, 2001.

Terezakis, Katie. *The Immanent Word: The Turn to Language in German Philosophy 1759–1801.* Routledge, 2007.

Trabant, Jürgen. "Herder's Discovery of the Ear." In *Herder Today: Contributions from the International Herder Conference,* ed. Kurt Mueller-Vollmer, 345–366. De Gruyter 1990.

von Uexküll, Jakob. "A Stroll through the Worlds of Animals and Men: A Picture Book of Invisible Worlds." *Semiotica* 89, no. 3–4 (1992): 319–391.

Vetlesen, Arne Johan. *A Philosophy of Pain,* trans. John Irons. Reaktion Books, 2009.

Weissberg, Liliane. "Language's Wound: Herder, Philoctetes, and the Origin of Speech." *Modern Language Notes* 104, no. 3 (1989): 548–579.

Wellbery, David. *Lessing's Laocoon: Semiotics and Aesthetics in the Age of Reason.* Cambridge University Press, 1984.

Wellbery, David. *The Specular Moment: Goethe's Early Lyric and the Beginnings of Romanticism.* Stanford University Press, 1996.

Wilson, Edmund. "Philoctetes: The Wound and the Bow." In *The Wound and the Bow: Seven Studies in Literature,* 272–295. Houghton Mifflin, 1941.

Winckelmann, Johann Joachim. *Reflections on the Imitation of Greek Works in Painting and Sculpture*, trans. Henry Fusseli. London, 1765.

Winckelmann, Johann Joachim. "Winckelmann's Remarks on the Laököon" [passages from *Geschichte der Kunst des Alterthums*], trans. E. S. Morgan. *Journal of Speculative Philosophy* 2, no.4 (1869): 213–215.

Wittgenstein, Ludwig. *The Blue and Brown Books: Preliminary Studies for the "Philosophical Investigations."* Harper & Row, 1960.

Wittgenstein, Ludwig. *On Certainty*, ed. G. E. M. Anscombe and G. H. Wright. Harper Torch Books, 1972.

Wittgenstein, Ludwig. *Philosophical Investigations*, 4th ed., trans. G. E. M. Anscombe, P. M. S. Hacker, and J. Schulte. Blackwell. 2009.

Woolf, Virginia. *On Being Ill: Notes from Sick Rooms*. Paris Press, 2002.

Woolf, Virginia. *The Waves*. Harvest Books, 1978.

Zuckert, Rachel. "Sculpture and Touch: Herder's Aesthetics of Sculpture." *Journal of Aesthetics and Art Criticism* 67, no. 3 (2009): 285–299.

INDEX